Clinical Microbiology

Laboratory Manual
and Workbook

With Colour Plates

W0234563

Student's Name:..

Roll No.: .... Year/Session: ....

University Roll No.: ....

Name of the Course: ....

Name of the Institution:..

This is to certify that this is a bonafide practical work done by ....
during the year 20___ – 20___. His/her work is complete/incomplete/excellent/
satisfactory/good/fair.

Signature of Staff in-charge
Signature of Prof. & HOD

Submitted for University Examination in the year_____

Examiners:_____   _____

Clinical Microbiology

Laboratory Manual and Workbook

With Colour Plates

Bani Baral MSc, PhD
Officiating Principal
Integrated Institute of Technology
Dwarka, New Delhi

Anandita Mandal MBBS, MD
Ex Director-Professor
Department of Microbiology
GB Pant Hospital, New Delhi

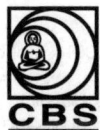

CBS Publishers & Distributors Pvt Ltd

New Delhi • Bengaluru • Chennai • Kochi • Mumbai • Pune
Hyderabad • Kolkata • Nagpur • Patna • Vijayawada

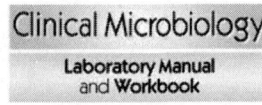

ISBN: 978-81-239-2519-6

Copyright © Authors and Publisher

First Edition: 2015

Published by Satish Kumar Jain and produced by Varun Jain for

CBS Publishers & Distributors Pvt Ltd

4819/XI Prahlad Street, 24 Ansari Road, Daryaganj, New Delhi 110 002, India.

Ph: 23289259, 23266861, 23266867   Website: www.cbspd.com

Fax: 011-23243014   e-mail: delhi@cbspd.com; cbspubs@airtelmail.in.

Corporate Office: 204 FIE, Industrial Area, Patparganj, Delhi 110 092

Ph: 4934 4934   Fax: 4934 4935   e-mail: publishing@cbspd.com; publicity@cbspd.com

Branches

- **Bengaluru:** Seema House 2975, 17th Cross, K.R. Road,
  Banasankari 2nd Stage, Bengaluru 560 070, Karnataka
  Ph: +91-80-26771678/79   Fax: +91-80-26771680   e-mail: bangalore@cbspd.com
- **Chennai:** 7, Subbaraya Street, Shenoy Nagar, Chennai 600 030, Tamil Nadu
  Ph: +91-44-26260666, 26208620   Fax: +91-44-42032115   e-mail: chennai@cbspd.com
- **Kochi:** Ashana House, No. 39/1904, AM Thomas Road, Valanjambalam, Eranakulam 682 018, Kochi Kerala
  Ph: +91-484-4059061-65   Fax: +91-484-4059065   e-mail: kochi@cbspd.com
- **Mumbai:** 83-C, Dr E Moses Road, Worli, Mumbai-400018, Maharashtra
  Ph: +91-22-24902340/41   Fax: +91-22-24902342   e-mail: mumbai@cbspd.com
- **Pune:** Bhuruk Prestige, Sr. No. 52/12/2+1+3/2 Narhe, Haveli
  (Near Katraj-Dehu Road Bypass), Pune 411 041, Maharashtra
  Ph: +91-20-64704058, 64704059, 32392277 Fax: +91-20-24300160   e-mail: pune@cbspd.com

Representatives

- **Hyderabad** 0-9885175004
- **Nagpur** 0-9021734563
- **Kolkata** 0-9831437309, 0-9051152362
- **Patna** 0-9334159340
- **Vijayawada** 0-9000660880

Printed at: Goyal Offset

Preface

Science students spend a considerable part of their practical classes preparing their laboratory files/notebooks copying the handwritten practical instructions. Besides the possibility of incorrect copying of instruction materials, time for their hands-on training gets reduced defeating the very purpose of conducting the practical classes.

This workbook is intended to be a replacement of the instructions given in the existing practical files/journals of clinical microbiology students so as to enable them to devote quality time towards their assigned work in the practical classes.

We acknowledge the sources of instructions and illustrations used in this compilation. Most of them are listed in the references.

We are grateful to Mr YN Arjuna, Senior Vice President, CBSPD, for his encouragement, and to his full team for extending all the cooperation to make this book compilation possible.

We hope to receive the feedback and suggestions from the students and their mentors.

We dedicate this compilation to our parents.

Bani Baral
Anandita Mandal

Contents

Preface   v

Colour Plates 1–7   between pp 120 and 121

1. Introduction to a clinical microbiology laboratory   1

2. Importance of labels in a laboratory   11

3. Clinical laboratory safety   14

4. Preparation of cleaning agents and techniques of cleaning glassware   22

5. Packaging and preparation of materials for sterilization   29

6. Equipment used for sterilization   33

7. Sterilization of various articles   40

8. Different types of microscopes: Handling and care
   of bright field microscope   46

9. Examination of morphology of microorganisms under
   bright field microscope   55

10. Simple staining   59

11. Demonstration of bacterial motility by hanging drop method   62

12. Gram staining   65

13. Ziehl-Neelsen staining   70

14. Albert staining   76

15. Capsule staining   79

16. Preparation of various culture media   83

17. Cultivation of bacteria   93

18. Macroscopic examination of bacterial growth on liquid
    and solid medium   102

19. Study of biochemical activities of bacteria in culture medium   108

20. Testing antimicrobial susceptibility of bacteria: Kirby-Bauer method   129

21. Isolation and identification of pure bacterial cultures   135

22. General guidelines for collection and transport of clinical
    specimens for bacteriological examination   139

23. Route from patient to microbial diagnosis 142

24. Processing of urine samples for culture and antibiotic sensitivity 143

25. Processing of fecal sample for culture and sensitivity 147

26. Processing of pus sample for culture and sensitivity 152

27. Processing of throat swab and nasopharyngeal swab samples
    for culture and sensitivity 154

28. Processing of sputum sample for culture and sensitivity 158

29. Processing of blood sample for culture and sensitivity 163

30. Processing of cerebrospinal fluid sample for culture and sensitivity 167

31. Bacteriological examination of water, milk, food and air 173

32. Examination of stool for diagnosis of intestinal parasitic infection 184

33. Laboratory diagnosis of fungal infection 191

34. Antigen–antibody reactions 198

35. Enzyme-linked immunosorbent assay 208

36. Polymerase chain reaction technology 214

37. Automation in clinical microbiology laboratory 218

   Index 221

Introduction to a Clinical Microbiology Laboratory

1.1 AIM

To familiarize the students with a clinical microbiology laboratory.

1.2 LEARNING OUTCOME

After this orientation, the students learn the names of various equipment, apparatus and laboratory ware used in a clinical microbiology laboratory and the purpose for which these are used. They also learn to read and understand importance of labels on the equipment, laboratory ware, bottles of chemicals and on different kits.

1.3 LIST OF MACHINERY AND EQUIPMENT IN A CLINICAL MICROBIOLOGY LABORATORY

Advanced level clinical microbiology laboratories are automated.

Routine microbiology laboratories are equipped with all or most of the equipment listed as under:

Air conditioner	Hot air oven
Anaerobic jar	Hybridisation incubator
Autoclave	Incubator
Auto pipette	Inspissator
Balance: analytical, chemical, single pan	Magnetic stirrer with hot plate
Biological safety cabinet (BSC)	MacIntosh and Fildes' jar
Bunsen burner	Membrane filter assembly
Different types of centrifuge with extra heads/ rotors	Micropipette
	Microscope
Colony counter	Needle destroyer
Computer system with printer, UPS, etc.	pH meter
Desiccators	Pipette washer
Distilled water plant	Power supply units
Draining board with pegs	Refrigerator
Electrophoresis units	Slide warmer
ELISA reader	Smoke detector
Eye wash facility	Thermo cycler
First aid box	Transilluminator
Freezer	Vacuum pump
Fume hood	VDRL slide rotator
Gas pak system	Vortex mixer
Gas leakage detector	Water bath

Additional equipment may be procured as per requirement.

1.4 LIST OF GLASSWARE/PLASTICWARE

1. Beaker (with spout and without spout), with graduation or without graduation: capacity 50 ml, 100 ml, 250 ml, 500 ml, 1 liter and 2 liter (Fig. 1.1)
2. Bottle:

   Blood collection bottle: 100 ml, 250 ml and 500 ml

   Blood culture bottle 250 ml

   Dropping bottles (Fig. 1.3)

   Mc Cartney bottle: 210 ml, screw capped, flat bottom (Fig. 1.2)

   Reagent bottle (colourless), reagent bottle (amber coloured) narrow mouth and wide mouth: capacity 100 ml, 250 ml and 500 ml.
3. Cylinder (measuring): capacity 10 ml, 50 ml, 100 ml, 250 ml, 500 ml, 1 liter (Fig. 1.4)
4. Discarding jar for slides.
5. Erlenmeyer flask (conical, with rim and without rim): capacity 50 ml, 100 ml, 250 ml, 500 ml, 1 litre, 2 litre, 3 litre (Fig. 1.5).
6. Filtering flask: 500 ml, 1 litre (Fig. 1.6).
7. Funnel: diameter 25 mm, 50 mm, 75 mm, 100 mm.
8. Test tubes (with rim and without rim), heavy duty, autoclavable, with approximate length × outer diameter as under:
   - 18 cm × 1.5 cm (culture tubes).
   - 15 cm × 1.5 cm [for inspissating (thickening) serum, for making agar slant, for storage of media, for pouring plates and for holding swabs].
   - 7.5 × 1.2 cm (for carbohydrate utilization test).
   - Test tubes (rimless) with rubber stoppers (Fig. 1.7).
9. Centrifuge tube with stopper and without stopper (graduated, plain): 10 ml, 15 ml (Fig. 1.8).
10. Petri dish: diameters 100 mm, 150 mm, 200 mm (Fig. 1.9).
11. Pipette (graduated): 1 ml, 2 ml, 5 ml, and 10 ml (Figs 1.10 A and B).
12. Weighing bottles.

Additional laboratory ware may be procured according to their and specific requirement.

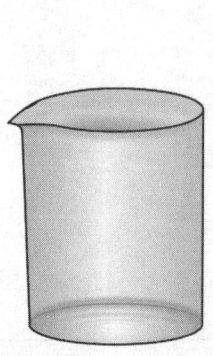

Fig. 1.1: Beaker with spout

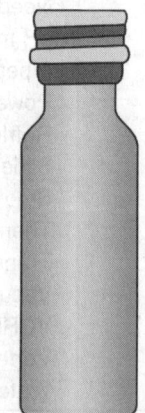

Fig. 1.2: McCartney bottle

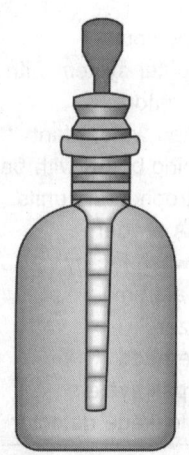

Fig. 1.3: Dropping bottle

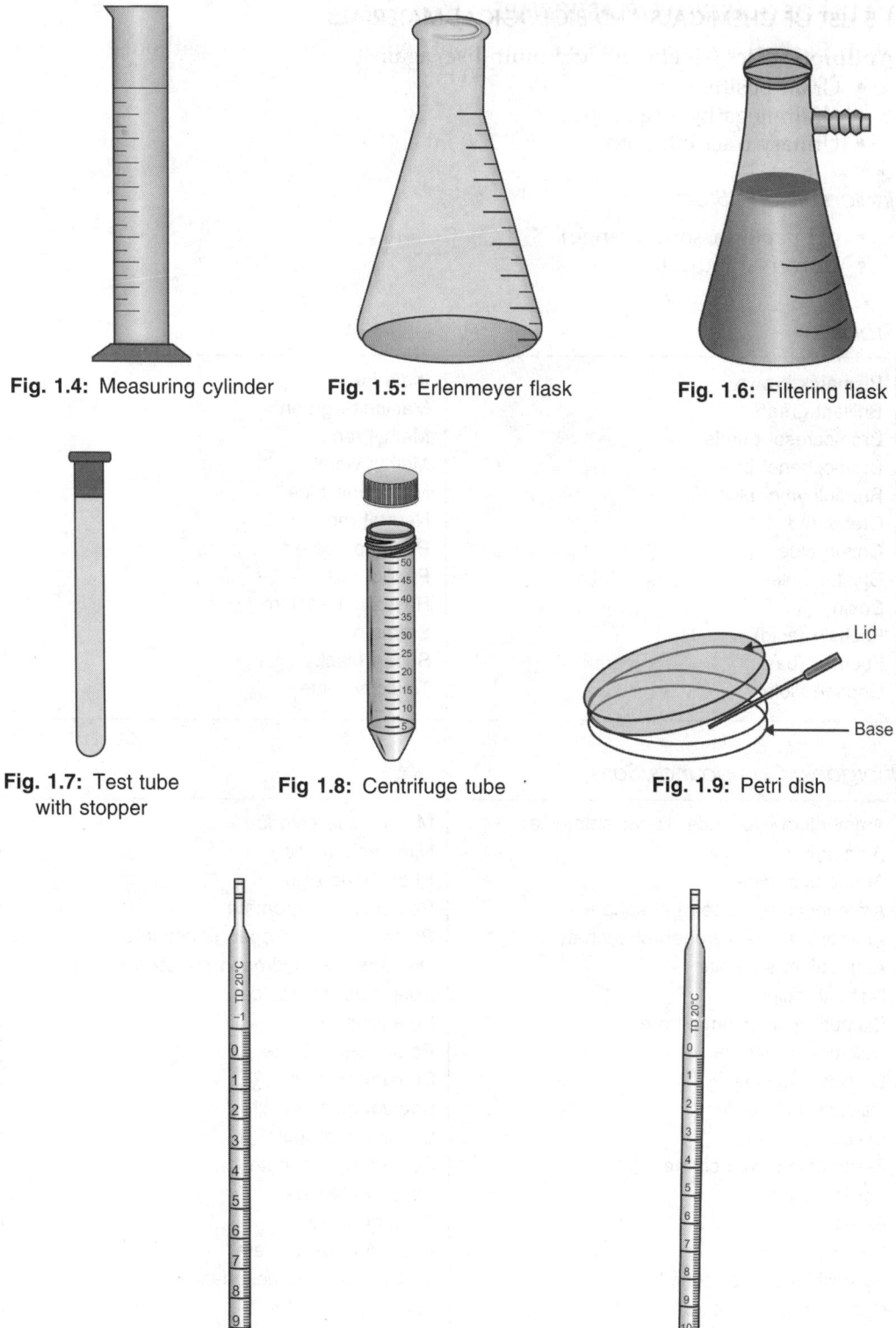

Fig. 1.4: Measuring cylinder   **Fig. 1.5:** Erlenmeyer flask   **Fig. 1.6:** Filtering flask

Fig. 1.7: Test tube with stopper   **Fig 1.8:** Centrifuge tube   **Fig. 1.9:** Petri dish

(A) Serological pipette (graduation continues till the tip)   (B) Mohr pipette (graduation ends before the tip)

Figs 1.10 A and B: Graduated pipettes

1.5 LIST OF CHEMICALS AND BIOLOGICAL MATERIALS

Antibiotic discs (single disc and multidisc) against

- Gram-positive cocci
- Gram-negative organisms
- Urinary tract infection

Indicators and Stains

- pH paper (assorted range)
- Universal indicator

Stains

Bismarck brown	India ink
Brilliant green	Malachite green
Bromocresol purple	Methyl red
Bromophenol blue	Methyl violet
Bromothymol blue	Methylene blue
Cresol red	Neutral red
Cotton blue	Phenolphthalein
Crystal violet	Phenol red
Eosin	Resazurin sodium
Fuchsin (acid)	Safranin
Fuchsin (basic)	Sudan black
Gentian violet	Toluidine blue

Inorganic Compounds/Salts

Ammonium hydroxide (liquor ammonia)	Manganese chloride
Ammonium chloride	Nitric acid (conc.)
Ammonium citrate	Phosphoric acid
Ammonium hydrogen phosphate	Potassium dichromate
Ammonium di -hydrogen phosphate	Potassium dihydrogen phosphate
Ammonium sulphate	Di-potassium hydrogen phosphate
Bismuth sulphite	Potassium hydroxide
Bismuth ammonium citrate	Potassium iodide
Calcium carbonate	Potassium tellurite
Calcium chloride	Sodium acetate
Calcium hydroxide	Sodium acid selenite
Copper sulphate	Sodium carbonate
Ferric ammonium citrate	Sodium bicarbonate
Ferric chloride	Sodium chloride
Ferric sulphate	Sodium citrate
Ferrous sulphate	Sodium deoxycholate
Hydrochloric acid (conc.)	Sodium glycerophosphate
Hydrogen peroxide	Sodium hydroxide
Iodine	Sodium hydrogen phosphate
Magnesium chloride	Sodium dihydrogen phosphate
Magnesium citrate	Sodium nitrate
Magnesium sulphate	Sodium nitrite

(Contd.)

Sodium pyruvate Sodium potassium tartrate Sodium sulphate Sodium thiosulphate	Sodium taurocholate Sulphuric acid (conc.) Zinc sulphate

Organic Compounds

Acid Acetic acid (Glacial) Ascorbic acid Benzoic acid Carbolic acid (phenol) Citric acid Lactic acid Oxalic acid Succinic acid Tartaric acid **Alcohol** Methyl alcohol Ethyl alcohol Propyl alcohol Butyl alcohol Amyl alcohol Isoamyl alcohol Glycerol **Carbohydrates** Arabinose Fructose Galactose Glucose Inulin	**Carbohydrates** Lactose Mannose Maltose Sucrose Xylose **Miscellaneous** Agar agar powder Alpha naphthol Benzidine Chloroform Creatine Cresol with soap solution Ether Formaldehyde Glycerol monoacetate Glucose 6 phosphate Para dimethyl aminobenzaldehyde Peptone Phenyl alanine Starch Tetramethyl paraphenylene diamine dihydrochloride Tween 20 Urea Xylene

Media/Miscellaneous Biological Items

Bacitracin disc Egg Deoxycholate citrate agar medium MacConkey agar medium Müller Hinton agar medium Minced meat Nutrient agar medium	Triple sugar iron medium Optochin discs Pancreatic extract Sterile sheep blood (from supplier) Urea broth Yeast Xylose lysine deoxycholate agar medium

Laboratory Kits for

Antistreptolysin O titre determination C-reactive protein titre determination Rheumatoid factor test VDRL test	Widal test ELISA test PCR reaction

Additional materials may be procured as per requirement

1.6 LIST OF MISCELLANEOUS ITEMS

Aluminium baskets (autoclavable, perforated): assorted sizes, with and without partitions.	Nichrome wire
Aluminium foil	Filter paper sheets
Band aid	Paraffin ring maker
Brown paper	Parafilm
Cavity slide	Pasteur pipettes
Capillaries	Pipette bulb/mechanical pipetting device
Cedar wood oil	Pipette washer
Cotton rolls absorbent	Pipette can for storing pasteur pipettes and other pipettes
Cotton rolls non-absorbent	Pipette stand
Cleaning brushes (assorted size)	Plasticin
Cleaning material—surf, vim, teepol	Preserved stained slides of different microorganisms
Containers for waste disposal with colour codes	Rubber gloves
Cover slip (blue star/standard make) boxes 22 mm × 22 mm, 24 mm × 24 mm	Rubber teats
Durham's tube	Rubber tubing
Duster	Slide boxes (blue star) plain
Discarding jars	Slide boxes with slides having frosted end at one side
Dustbin	Spatula
Enameled tray without lid 18" × 12", 12"× 8"	Spare eyepieces and objectives of microscopes
Enameled tray with lid 18" × 12", 12" × 8"	Specimen containers of assorted size
Filter paper box (Whatman) No. 1	Sticks for making swabs
First aid kits	Stirrer bar for magnetic stirrer (assorted size)
Face mask	Syringe with needles (19 G, 20G, 21G, 22G) 2 ml, 5 ml, 10 ml
Funnel stand	Stopwatch
Gas lighter	Test tube stands (assorted size)
Gauge pieces and gauge than (standard size)	Test tube holder
Glass rods	Tripod stand
Glass tubing	Thread ball
Gum paper	Tissue paper
Hand cleaner: savlon/dettol/lifebuoy, etc.	Tripod stand
Inoculating loop and loop holder	Wash bottle
Jug with lid	Waste paper baskets
Labels (self sticking)/glass marking pencil/permanent markers	Weighing paper
Lens cleaner	Weight box and fractional weights
Lens cleaning paper	Wire gauge
Membrane filter (for syringe and for filtering funnel)	

Additional materials may be procured as per specific requirement

1.7 STUDENTS ACTIVITY

Take a look at your microbiology laboratory and get familiar with available materials. Make a record as under:

1.7.1 Equipment Seen

Date	Name of the equipment	Use of the laboratory ware as explained	Teacher's signature

1.7.2 Laboratory Ware Seen

Date	Name of the laboratory ware	Use of the equipment as explained	Teacher's signature

1.7.3 Chemical Inventory

Date

Name of the chemical	Manufact-urer	Qty (pack)	Physical state		Hazard class as displayed on the package							Teacher's signature
			S	L	T	Co	F	Car	A	Cau	R	

S: Solid, L: Liquid, T: Toxic, Co: Corrosive, F: Flammable, Car: Carcinogenic, A: Acid, Cau: Caustic, R: Radioactive.

1.7.4 Miscellaneous Items/Apparatus/Tools Seen

Date	Name of the item	Use of the item as explained	Teacher's signature

2

Importance of Labels in a Laboratory

2.1 AIM

To educate the students the importance of labels in a laboratory.

2.2 LEARNING OUTCOME

The students understand the importance of labels on various articles, information available on the labels and also learn to label the materials prepared/used by them while working in the laboratory.

Labels are essential for proper identification of each item in the laboratory and their proper use. Labels may be written or printed or displayed as graphic matter affixed to or appearing upon the containers or outside package of the material.

2.3 LABEL ON AN INSTRUMENT

Label on an instrument should have following information on its surface/package.

- Name of the instrument.
- Model designation.
- Serial number.
- Immediate safety hazards to the operator, if any.
- Manufacturer/distributor's name and address.
- Electrical rating information, if applicable.

After receiving the instrument, record the name and phone number of the contact person for installation/future services. Check the package for the instruction manual and documents on guaranty/warrantee/maintenance.

2.4 LABEL ON CHEMICALS

Complete label on chemicals generally include the following information (Fig. 2.1 for a chemical)

- Product name (A in the Fig. 2.1)
- Principal use or intended use
- Cautionary statement/hazard classification (B in the Fig. 2.1)
- Name and address of the manufacturer, re-packager or distributor
- Catalogue number
- Lot or control number (C in the Fig. 2.1)
- Quantity of contents expressed in terms of number, mass, volume, concentration or other applicable quantity designation (D in the Fig. 2.1)
- Storage information.
- Expiry date.

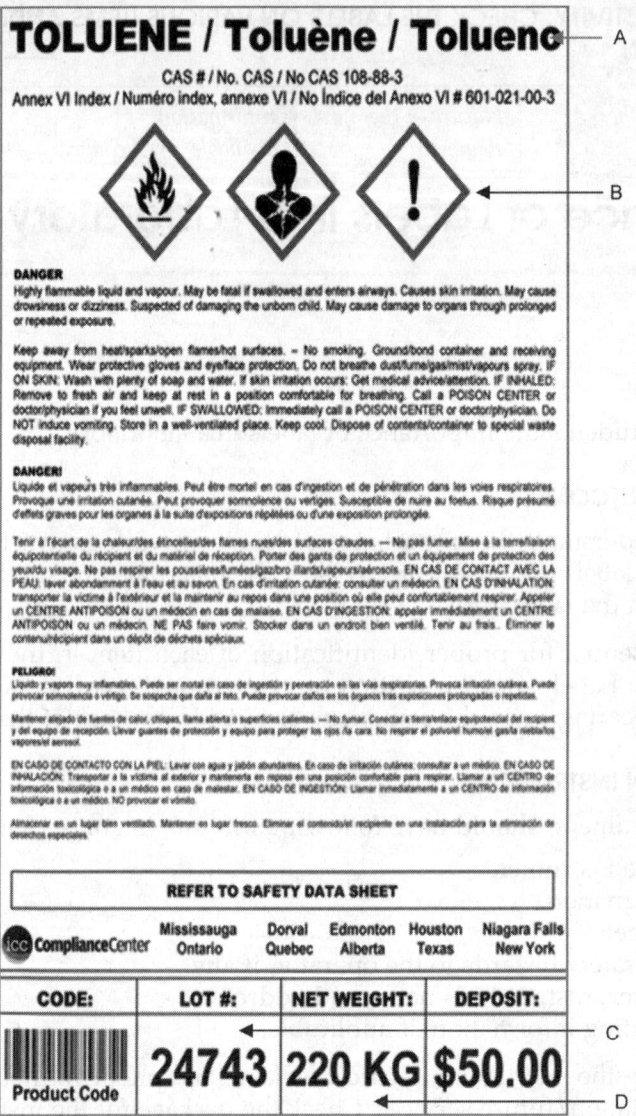

Fig. 2.1: Label on a chemical

2.5 LABELS ON THE LABORATORY PREPARED MATERIALS

Labels on the laboratory prepared materials are essential for correct identity and safe use of the material.

Minimum information on the label of the laboratory prepared materials must include the following

- Name of the material.
- Hazards, if applicable.
- Storage condition.
- Date of preparation.
- Expiry date.
- Name of the preparer.

2.6 STUDENT'S ACTIVITY: CHECK THE LABELS ON VARIOUS ITEMS AND RECORD YOUR OBSERVATION

Date	Name of the item seen	Nature of the item seen	Information available on the label	Teacher's signature

3

Clinical Laboratory Safety

3.1 AIM

To educate the students about different hazards present in the laboratory and importance of ensuring clinical laboratory safety.

3.2 LEARNING OUTCOME

The students can identify the potential hazards in the laboratory, become aware of essential elements required for ensuring laboratory safety and safety precautions to be taken at personal level.

3.3 ELEMENTS OF LABORATORY SAFETY

Elements required to ensure laboratory safety are

　　3.3.1: Facility design.

　　3.3.2: Availability of safety equipment.

　　3.3.3: Laboratory practice at the level of individual laboratory worker.

3.3.1 Facility Design

Components of facility design include:

- Availability of hand washing facility.
- Availability of decontamination facilities, e.g. autoclave.
- Proper interior of the laboratory.
- Separation of laboratory area from public access.
- Specialized ventilation system for environmental safety.

3.3.2 Availability of Safety Equipment

Safety equipment to be made available in a clinical microbiology laboratory are:

3.3.2.1 General Safety Equipment

General safety equipment in a clinical microbiology laboratory includes biohazard waste container, biosafety cabinets (BSC), eyewash stations, fire extinguisher, fire blankets, first aid equipment, fume hood, mechanical pipetting device, sharp container, etc.

3.3.2.2 Personal Protective Equipment (PPE)

Examples of personal protective equipment are laboratory coat, face shields, gloves, gown, eye shield, goggles, mask, vaccination, etc.

3.3.3 Laboratory Practice at the Level of the Individual Laboratory Worker

Each user of the laboratory facility must know the potential hazards present in a laboratory and must take careful measures for personal hygiene, cleanliness of the workplace, personal safety and safety of others while handling hazardous materials.

3.4 LABORATORY HAZARDS

The hazards in a clinical laboratory can be broadly classified as

- Physical hazards.
- Chemical and reagent hazards.
- Biological hazards.

3.4.1 Physical Hazards Encountered in a Microbiology Laboratory Include

3.4.1.1 Electrical Hazards

Electrical hazards may arise due to accidental or unexpected starting of electrical equipment, presence of open live wiring or fire hazard due to short circuit. Moreover, many electrical devices are also potential ignition sources.

Electrical hazards may result in:
- **Direct injuries** a such as electrical burns, thermal contact burns and
- **Indirect injuries** from involuntary muscle contractions from the electric shock (Fig. 3.1).

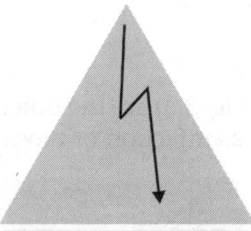

Fig. 3.1: Graphic display of electrical hazard (shock hazard)

3.4.1.2 Mechanical Hazards

Mechanical hazards are mostly related to mishandling of equipment/various tools or glassware or the possibility of tripping in a cluttered laboratory. Mechanical hazards can cause various degree of physical injury.

3.4.1.3 Fire Hazards

Fire hazards may be caused due to open flame, electrical short circuit, electrical overloading and improper storage of flammable chemicals, etc.

3.4.2 Chemical and Reagent Hazards

Chemicals may be toxic (e.g. acryl amide), corrosive/caustic (e.g. sodium hydroxide), flammable (e.g. ether), carcinogenic (e.g. benzidine), explosive (e.g. metallic sodium), irritant (e.g. formaldehyde).

In Figure 3.2 depicts the labeling of chemicals according to the old symbols and the globally harmonised system (GHS) pictogram.

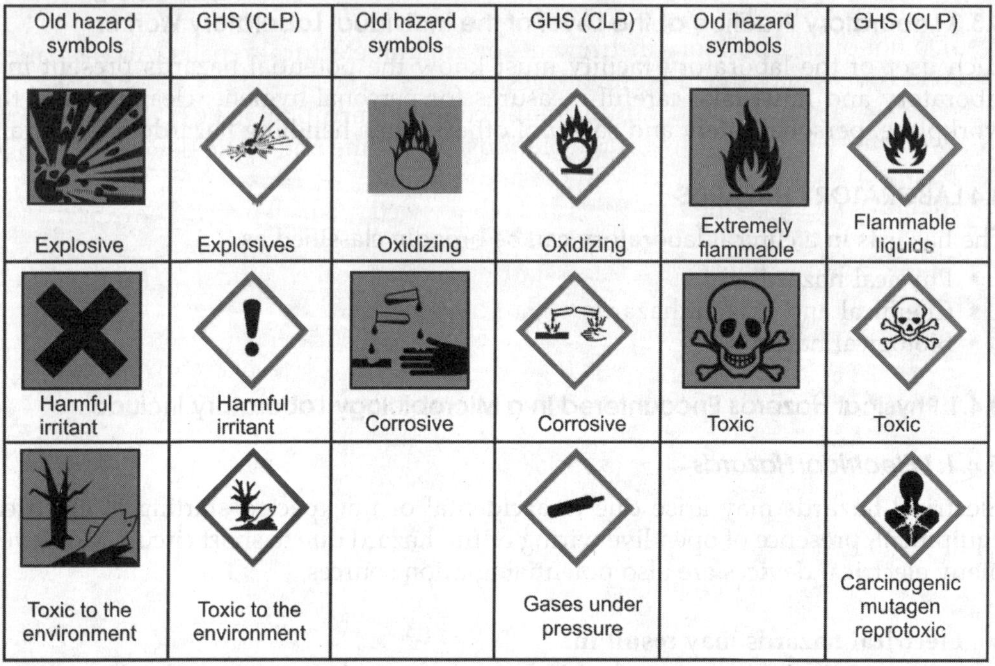

Old hazard symbols	GHS (CLP)	Old hazard symbols	GHS (CLP)	Old hazard symbols	GHS (CLP)
Explosive	Explosives	Oxidizing	Oxidizing	Extremely flammable	Flammable liquids
Harmful irritant	Harmful irritant	Corrosive	Corrosive	Toxic	Toxic
Toxic to the environment	Toxic to the environment		Gases under pressure		Carcinogenic mutagen reprotoxic

Fig. 3.2: Chemical hazard symbols, old and new

You must make yourself familiar with the symbols on the label of the chemical you are using by referring to Fig. 3.2.

3.4.3 Biological Hazards

Biological hazards (displayed at Fig. 3.3) are the potentially infective materials present in the laboratory resulting in cross infection or cross contamination.

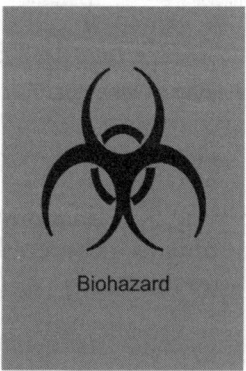

Biohazard

Fig. 3.3: Graphic display of biohazard

3.5 PREVENTIVE MEASURES AGAINST LABORATORY HAZARDS

3.5.1 Preventive Measures Against Physical Hazards

3.5.1.1 Precautions Against Electrical Hazards

- Carefully read and follow all operating instructions of the manufacturer's manual and electrical codes before installing and operating new equipment.

- Do not open laboratory instruments or attempt electrical repairs. Access panels and covers may shield high voltages.
- Use extra caution and ground fault circuit interrupter (GFCI) devices when working with wet hands, salt solutions, and some anti-static devices that may enhance electrical contact with the body.
- Remove metallic rings, watches and other jewelry, which may become part of an electrical circuit when working with electrical devices.
- Avoid accidental or unexpected starting of electrical equipment. This can cause severe injury-even death.
- Never store flammable liquids near the electrical devices that are potential ignition sources.
- Ensure that access to electric panels is un-obstructed and that each panel has necessary circuit breakers.
- Check for any spark at the time of operation.
- Disconnect the equipment from the power supply even for doing minor activities like changing microscope lamp, etc.
- Check the wires of the plug and cord for any exposed wire.
- Avoid using extension cords unless there is emergency.
- In case there is electric spark, remove the plug from the socket.
- In case of fire due to short circuit, switch off the mains immediately.
- Remove live electric wire only after taking proper safety measures, e.g. with a wooden rod, wearing rubber, gloves, etc.
- Always keep rubber mat/wooden planks under feet while carrying out electric repair.

3.5.1.2 Precautions Against Mechanical Hazards

- Install and operate all equipment according to the manufacturer's instructions.
- Use personal protective equipment.
- Avoid cluttering of the work area.

3.5.1.3 Precautions Against Fire Hazard

- Wear properly fitted cotton clothing without any loose ends and keep your hair pinned to avoid catching of the flame of Bunsen burner.
- Avoid conditions leading to fire due to short circuit.
- Check the efficacy date of fire safety equipment from time to time. Be familiar with the location of the fire exits in the building.

3.5.2. Precautions Against Chemical Hazards

- Use gowns, gloves, etc. before handling the chemical.
- Read the label on the chemical carefully. Handle the material as indicated in the label.
- Use a fume hood while working with flammable and volatile chemicals.
- Always use mechanical pipetting device.
- Never heat a tightly closed container. If a burner is used, distribute the heat with ceramic-centered wire gauze.
- Store the flammable and volatile chemicals in a well-ventilated area.
- Recap all reagent bottles containing toxic substances.
- Label hazardous chemicals appropriately indicating their proper storage, handling and disposal.

3.5.3 Precautions Against Biological Hazard

Treat all human blood and other human body fluids as if they were known to be infectious. Adopt universal precautions.

3.5.3.1 Practice of Universal Precautions Includes

- Always cover cuts and abrasions, if any on your body, with a waterproof dressing.
- Wear gloves during contact with body fluids, non-intact skin and mucous membranes. Never touch a wet specimen without gloves.
- Always wash your hands after removing the gloves.
- Wear personal protection equipment (PPE) especially if blood or other body fluids is likely to splash or spray. Use a mask and eye protection for protection of moist areas of your eyes, nose and mouth.
- Prevent two-handed recapping of needles.
- Use sharp items with utmost care. Safely collect needles and sharps (scalpel blades, lancets, razors, scissors, etc.), and dispose them in puncture and leak proof safety boxes.
- Perform all procedures with aseptic precautions.
- Clean up spills of blood and other body fluids promptly and carefully with disinfectant.
- Use certified biological safety cabinets (Class I, II, or III) and other physical containment devices like centrifuge safety cups, sealed centrifuge rotors, and containment caging for animals for all activities with materials that pose a threat of exposure to droplets, splashes, spills, or aerosols. Never use open bench while working with potentially infectious materials.
- **No mouth pipetting**; always use mechanical pipetting device.
- Do not wear protective clothing outside of the work area. Decontaminate the protective clothing before sending it for laundry.
- Use a safe system for health care waste management and disposal.
- Do not eat, drink or store any food material in the laboratory.
- Get yourself vaccinated against various infectious diseases.

3.5.3.2 Post-exposure Precautions

Type of exposure	Precaution
Needle stick or other sharp injury	Immediately wash the area with soap and water
Splash of body fluids/blood on eyes, nose or mouth	Immediately flush the area with water or saline
Splash of body fluids/blood on skin	Immediately flush the area with water or soap
Splash of culture	Immediately flush the area with antiseptic solution, soap and water

3.6 USE OF BIOLOGICAL SAFETY CABINETS

3.6.1 Principle of Working of a Biological Safety Cabinet

Biological safety cabinets (BSCs) use high efficiency particulate air (HEPA) filters to filter the air generated within the cabinet to provide protection of the worker, the immediate environment and the research material from infectious aerosols.

Depending on their construction, biological safety cabinets are classified as class I, class II or class III biosafety cabinet.

Class I BSC is a ventilated cabinet for **protection of personnel and environment. It has an un-recirculated inward airflow away from the operator** that exhausts all air to the atmosphere after filtration through a HEPA filter. **Class I cabinets are suitable for work where no product protection is required.**

Class II BSC is a ventilated cabinet for **protection of personnel, product, and environment.** It has an open front with inward airflow for personnel protection, downward HEPA filtered laminar airflow for product protection, and HEPA filtered exhausted air for environmental protection (Fig. 3.4).

Class III BSC is a totally enclosed, ventilated cabinet **of leak proof construction. Operations in the cabinet are conducted through attached rubber gloves.** The cabinet is maintained under negative air pressure. Air is drawn into the cabinet through HEPA filters. The **exhaust air is treated by double HEPA filtration or by HEPA filtration and air incineration.**

3.6.2 Parts of a Biological Safety Cabinet (Fig. 3.4)

Basic structure of a biological safety cabinet consists of following parts:

1. Front opening (A in Fig. 3.4)
2. Sash/night door (B in Fig. 3.4)
3. Exhaust HEPA filter (C in Fig. 3.4)
4. Supply HEPA filter (D in Fig. 3.4)
5. Rear plenum (E in Fig. 3.4)
6. Fan/blower unit (F in Fig. 3.4)
7. Chemical and fire resistant work surface (G in Fig. 3.4)
8. Base assembly with feet or castor (H in Fig. 3.4)

In addition to above basic structures, there are provisions for adequate lighting for optimum visibility of the work area, gas tap, vacuum tap, and UV light, etc. inside the cabinet and also the electrical sockets and manometer outside the cabinet.

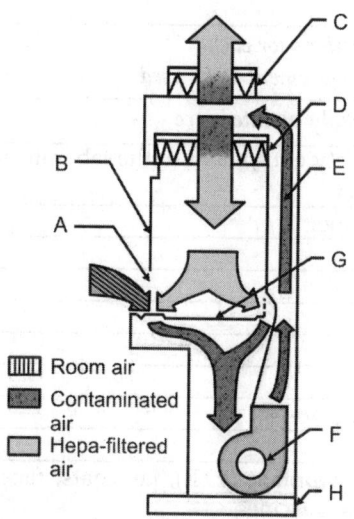

Fig. 3.4: Parts of a biological safety cabinet indicating flow of air

3.6.3 Operation of Biological Safety Cabinet

1. Carefully read the user's manual and familiarize yourself with the BSC before use.
2. Before working with a BSC, turn on the blowers and allow the blowers to run for approximately 5 minutes for proper pressures to build up.
3. Wear lab coats and appropriate gloves fitting over the cuffs of the coat.
4. Wash hands and arms before putting them inside the cabinet. Also remove any jewelry from the hands and wrists.
5. Adjust the stool to a proper height.
6. Wipe down all required materials with 70% ethanol before bringing them inside the cabinet. Gather all of them at once (in order to eliminate the number of entries into the BSC.)
7. Keep your hands within the clean area of the cabinet as much as possible. Do not touch your hair, face or clothing. Perform all work at a distance of minimum six inches from the front edge of the work surface to avoid contamination with outside air.
8. Maintain a direct path between the HEPA filter and the area inside the cabinet where the procedures are being performed. The hands must never obstruct airflow.
9. Always minimize clutter. Arrange objects in a manner to get full benefit of the laminar flow of air.
10. Avoid spraying solutions onto the HEPA filter or keeping objects touching the HEPA filter.
11. Clean the work surface of the biological safety cabinet thoroughly with alcohol in case something is spilled. Use a long side to side motion starting at the back of the cabinet and then working forward. Periodically clean the acrylic plastic sides.
12. Do not talk, cough or sneeze into the hood.
13. Every time after finishing the work, pull the shutter down and switch on the UV light to decontaminate the internal air.

3.7 LABORATORY RECORD

3.7.1 Complete the Following Check List for Your Laboratory

		Yes	No
Date	*Checked the electrical connections for each electrically operated gadget/equipment to be used*		
	Checked the equipment for daily maintenance		
	Availability of general safety equipment in the laboratory • Biological safety cabinet		
	• Biohazard waste container		
	• Eye wash station		
	• Fire blankets		
	• Fire extinguisher		
	• First aid box		
	• Fumehood		
	• Mechanical pipetting device		
	• Needle destroyer, etc.		
	• Personal protective equipment (PPE), i.e. coats, face shields, gloves, gowns, goggles, vaccines		
	• Sharp disposal container		

3.7.2 Make a Record Regarding Specific Precautions Taken by you While Handling Various Hazards in the Following Format

Date	Name of the item handled	Nature of hazard			Precautions taken	Teacher's signature
		Physical	*Chemical*	*Biological*		

Preparation of Cleaning Agents and Techniques of Cleaning Glassware

4.1 AIM

To familiarize the students with the names of different cleaning agents used for cleaning laboratory ware, their preparation and methods for cleaning of various laboratory ware.

4.2 LEARNING OUTCOME

Students learn to prepare the cleaning agents with due precautions and store them suitably after proper labeling. They are able to wash specific kinds of glass ware and store them properly.

4.3 GENERAL PROPERTIES OF A GOOD CLEANING AGENT

- It should soften water.
- It should not contain free alkali.
- It should be readily and completely soluble in warm water and should not precipitate in hot water or in cold water.
- It should have good wetting ability.
- It should be rinsed easily.
- It should be non-irritating to the hands.

For preparing cleaning agents, use soft water.

4.4 PREPARATION OF DIFFERENT CLEANING AGENTS

Ingredients/composition of various cleaning agents, their preparation and specific use are given in Table 4.1 along with relevant remarks.

4.5 TECHNIQUES OF CLEANING LABORATORY WARE

Cleaning of the laboratory ware is aimed at removing soil, dirt and various inorganic or organic materials from the laboratory ware.

General Conditions

- While cleaning laboratory ware, always use personal protective equipment/ materials.
- Select appropriate brushes for the shape and size of the laboratory ware. Brushes must be in good condition to avoid any abrasion of the glassware.

Table 4.1: Preparation and use of different cleaning agents

Name of the cleaning agent	Preparation of the cleaning agent	Used for	Special remarks
Commercial soap/ detergent	Dissolve required quantity in hot water.	General cleaning.	
Weak solution of **sodium carbonate**	Dissolve 0.5 to 1.0 g of sodium carbonate in 100 ml of warm water.	Removal of grease.	
1% Hydrochloric acid (HCl)	Add 2.7 ml of concentrated hydrochloric acid to 97.3 ml of water for making 100 ml (W/V) Add 1 ml HCl to 99 ml water (v/V).	Soaking new glassware for several hours before washing.	(Commercial concentrated hydrochloric acid is 12 M, 37% w/V)
1% Nitric acid	Add 1.5 ml conc nitric acid to 98.5 ml water to make 100 ml(w/V). Add 1 ml nitric acid to 99 ml water (v/V).		(Commercial nitric acid is 14M, 65% w/V)
6 M Hydrochloric acid	Add 50 ml of conc HCl to 50 ml of water to make 100 ml of 6M HCl.	Removing contaminants such as metallic compounds or organic materials other than grease.	This solution can cause severe burns
Base bath	Make saturated sodium hydroxide or potassium hydroxide solution in ethanol, methanol or isopropanol.	Cleaning of cloudy glassware with organic contaminants.	The base bath will react with skin. Alcohols are flammable.
Aquaregia	Mix 1 part concentrated HNO_3 and 3 parts conc HCl for storage, 1part H_2O may be added to the aquaregia to minimize generation of chlorine.	Very aggressive cleaning.	This is an extremely powerful oxidizing solution. It causes severe tissue damage. Clean the glassware and rinse thoroughly with water after taking out of aquaregia.
Acidic peroxide solution	Add 50 ml conc. sulphuric acid to 50 ml 3% hydrogen peroxide to make 100 ml **Or** Dissolve 36 g $(NH_4)_2S_2O_8$ (ammonium peroxy.	Specific removal of heavy precipitates that cannot be removed by ordinary cleaning agents	The H_2O_2/H_2SO_4 solution is both a strong oxidizing agent and a strong reducing agent, so care must be taken when using it.

Table 4.1: Preparation and use of different cleaning agents *(Contd.)*

Name of the cleaning agent	Preparation of the cleaning agent	Used for	Special remarks
	disulfate) in 2.2 litre of 98% H_2SO_4 (can be made right in the bottle of H_2SO_4, if the bottle is loosely stoppered.		
Chromic acid	Make a thin paste of 20 grams of fine powder of sodium dichromate or potassium dichromate with water in a 1 litre beaker. Slowly add approximately 300 ml of commercial concentrated sulfuric acid, stirring well. Transfer to a glass-stoppered bottle. Use the clear supernatant solution.	Not recommended	High-valent chromium is carcinogenic, teratogenic and causes severe environmental damage, the use of chromic acid is not recommended

4.5.1 Pre-cleaning Treatment of the Glassware

- Before washing, soak new glassware for several hours in acid water (1% solution of hydrochloric acid or nitric acid)
- Sterilize glassware which is contaminated with blood clots, culture media, etc. before cleaning.
- Before cleaning, disassemble the assembled glassware. De-grease the glassware's ground glass joints by boiling in a weak solution of sodium carbonate or by wiping them with a paper towel soaked in a small amount of fat solvent, e.g. ether, acetone or other solvents.

4.5.2 Cleaning Procedure

Cleaning of glassware, for which a simple solvent rinse is not sufficient, involves three steps.

1. Soaking
2. Washing and cleaning
3. Rinsing

4.5.2.1 Soaking

Place the glassware in a warm concentrated aqueous solution of a good non-abrasive detergent. Soak the glassware in cleaning solution for 20 – 30 minutes.

4.5.2.2 Washing and Cleaning

Soak the cleaning brush in a non-abrasive detergent solution. To remove the dirt, brush the inside and outside the glassware.

4.5.2.3 Rinsing

Rinse the glassware thoroughly with tap water and give a final rinse with distilled water. Ensure that all detergents or other cleaning fluids are removed from glassware. The water sheets off the clean glass.

4.6 DRYING GLASSWARE

You may dry the glassware by using any of the following methods:

- Place them on the drying rack with wooden pegs or invert them on a paper towel in baskets with their mouths downward and allow them to dry in the air.
- Place them in the drying oven (for items that are water-wet only, no flammable solvents) at a temperature not exceeding 140°C.
- Rinse with a solvent such as acetone, methanol or ethanol and then gently blow compressed air into the vessel until it is dry.

4.7 STORAGE

- Protect clean glassware from dust by plugging with cotton, by corking, by taping a heavy piece of paper over the mouth or by placing the glassware in a dust-free cabinet.
- Store glassware in specially designed racks. Avoid breakage by keeping individual pieces separated.

4.8 CLEANING OF SPECIFIC GLASSWARE

4.8.1 Used Pipettes

- Immediately after use, place pipettes, tips down, in a cylinder or tall jar of water. Place a pad of cotton or glass wool at the bottom of the jar to prevent breaking of the tips. An automatic pipette washer may be used in laboratories where a large number of pipettes are used daily.
- Ensure that the water level is high enough to immerse each pipette.
- At a convenient time, drain the pipettes and place them in another cylinder or jar containing dissolved detergent or a suitable cleaning solution.
- After soaking for several hours (mostly overnight), drain the pipettes.
- Run tap water over and through the pipettes until all traces of dirt are removed.
- Soak the pipettes in distilled water for at least one hour. Remove the pipettes from the distilled water.
- Dry the outside with a cloth, shake out the water from inside and dry in air or in electrically heated metallic pipette drier.
- After drying, place pipettes in a dust-free drawer.

4.8.2 Used Culture Tubes

- Sterilize the used culture tubes by autoclaving for 30 minutes at 121°C (15 lb pressure). Use of separate autoclave (earmarked for this) is advisable. Pour out the molten media while the tubes are hot.
- After the tubes are emptied, brush with detergent and water.
- Rinse thoroughly with tap water.
- Rinse with distilled water.
- Place in a basket and dry.

4.8.3 Serological Tubes

- If the tubes contain blood clots, discard the clots in a waste container. Place the tubes in a large basket.
- Put the basket in a large bucket or boiler. Cover with water, add appropriate quantity of soft soap or detergent and boil for 30 minutes.

- Clean with brush and rinse the tubes to remove all acid, alkali and detergent completely. Presence of traces of acid and alkali may destroy complement or may produce hemolysis. Detergents interfere with serologic reactions.
- Dry with the usual precautions.

Use serological tubes and other glassware for serological procedures only. Keep them separate from all other glassware.

4.8.4 Dishes and Culture Bottles

First sterilize the used petri dishes and culture bottles and then clean as detailed above under culture tubes.

4.8.5 Slides and Cover Slips

Always ensure that microscope slides and cover glass used for the preparation of blood films or bacteriologic smears are perfectly clean and free from scratches.

- Take four 1000 ml beakers (for slides) and four 250 ml beakers (for cover slips).
- Permanently mark one of each size beaker for liquid soap solution and one for alcohol solution. The other two beakers will be used exclusively for the rinsing procedures. Cover beakers with parafilm to prevent dust settling in them. Store glassware covered and dust free (Fig. 4.1).

4.8.5.1 Wash Process

1. Fill the 250 ml beaker (for cover slips) and the 1000 ml beaker (for slides) with water to the 50–75 ml level (for cover slip) or to 400–500 ml (for slides) respectively. Heat on the hot plate to just below the boiling point. Add 1/4 capful liquid concentrate soap for coverslips or 1/2 capful for slides.
2. Wear gloves and use forceps for handling slides and cover slips. Touch only the edges of the cover slips (or slides) with gloves and hold them at a corner. Be sure not to scratch surfaces.
3. **Place the cover slips** (or slides) in the beaker containing soap solution **one at a time.**
4. Very gently rub each coverslip/slide between your thumb and forefinger.

4.8.5.2 Rinse Process

1. Pour soap solution out of the beaker.
2. Fill the first rinse beaker with tap water above the material (cover slips or slides). Rinse the inside of the beaker as you fill it.
3. Swirl gently for 1 to 2 minutes. Do not shake as this may scratch surfaces.
4. Pour water out.
5. Repeat this washing many times to get rid of the soap completely.
6. Fill the second rinse beaker with de-ionized water and transfer the cover slips or slides **one at a time** into the new beaker.
7. Tilt the beaker so that the cover slips/slides stand on edge and lean against the wall of the beaker. This position will facilitate their removal with forceps.
8. Pour water out of beaker and continue rinsing 4 times.
9. Fill alcohol beaker with 80% ethyl alcohol and place cover slip/slide one at a **time** into the beaker. Using gloves and forceps, touch only the edges of the coverslips or slides (Fig. 4.1).

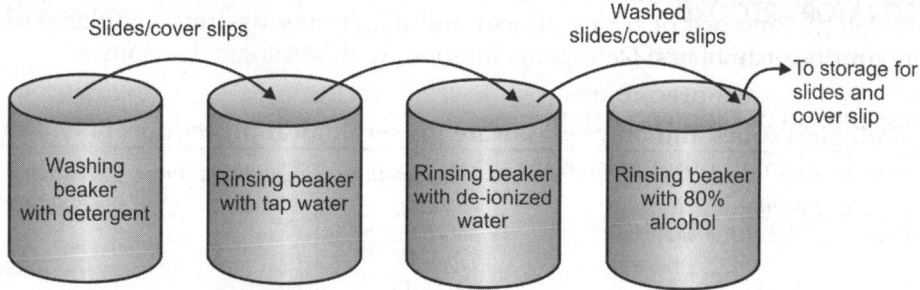

Fig. 4.1: Washing of used slides or coverslips

4.8.5.3 Drying and Storage

Remove one cover slip at a time with dried forceps and replace them in their original box and cover. For protection against dust, store the cleaned slides between two layers of lens tissue at the top and bottom of the box.

Soaking Materials for Different Classes of Plasticware

Plasticware made of **Polyolefins** and **fluorinated hydrocarbons** [(low-density polyethylene (LDPE), high-density polyethylene (HDPE), fluorinated polyethylene (FLPE), polypropylene (PP), polymethyl pentene (PMP), polytetrafluoroethylene (PTFE), polyfluoroalcoxy (PFA), fluorinated ethylene propylene (FEP), ethylene-tetrafluoroethylene (ETFE), ethylene-chloro trifluoro-ethylene copolymer (E-CTFE)].

For all these materials with slight contamination, use a chemically neutral (pH 7) cleaning agent. For removal of heavy contamination, use an alkaline cleaning agent.

Plasticware made of Polycarbonate

Use only pH 7 neutral cleaning agents. Use only alcohol as solvent to remove grease and oil. Other solvents attack these plastics. Do not use alkaline cleaning agents.

Plasticware made of Polystyrene

Use neutral cleaning agents only. Use only alcohols as solvent to remove grease and oils. Do not autoclave under any condition.

Plasticware made of Polysulphonate

Never use cleaning agents containing Tween.

4.9 CLEANING METHODS FOR PLASTICWARE

1. Take containers made of moulded plastic or pyrex glass that has a loose fitting lid.
2. Fill the container with a solution of 1M nitric acid or an appropriate soaking material.
3. Allow the plasticware to soak overnight for mild contamination. Keep in bath for about one week for heavy contamination. Use a pair of tongs to sink the plasticware in the cleaning solution.
4. Take the cleaned plasticware off the bath, rinse with distilled water and put to dry.
5. Place in the drier at low temperature.

4.10 LABORATORY RECORD

Maintain your records as under:

4.10.1 Preparation of Cleaning Agent

Date	Name of the cleaning agent prepared	Volume of the cleaning material prepared	Whether the cleaning solutions labeled properly	Condition for storage	Teacher's signature

4.10.2 Cleaning of Glassware/Plasticware

Date	Type and no. of each type of laboratory ware cleaned	Cleaning material(s) used	Drying method used	Teacher's signature

5

Packaging and Preparation of Materials for Sterilization

5.1 AIM

To educate the students the importance of plugging/wrapping of various articles before sterilization.

5.2 LEARNING OUTCOME

The students understand that before sterilization of the articles, plugging/wrapping of materials is essential in order to prevent recontamination of the sterilized articles. They also learn the techniques of plugging/packing of various articles.

5.3 PURPOSE OF PACKAGING

Packaging or plugging is done before sterilization
- for articles that can be re-used,
- to allow sterilization of the packaged/plugged articles,
- to maintain sterility of contents until the package/plug is opened, and,
- to permit delivery of contents without contamination.

5.4 PACKAGING MATERIALS (STERILIZATION WRAPS)

The choice of packaging systems includes:
- **Non-absorbent cotton wool**
- **Woven fabrics**, usually 100 percent cotton, cotton polyester blends and synthetic blends, either treated or untreated.
- **Non-woven materials** made of plastic polymers, cellulose fibres, aluminium foil or washed paper pulp bonded under pressure into sheets.
- **Peel pouches** made of a variety of materials, including paper, cellophane, polyethylene, and various paper-plastic combinations.
- **Rigid container systems** which are specially designed metal or plastic containers for holding the articles.

5.5 PROCEDURE FOR WRAPPING OF LABORATORY WARE BEFORE STERILIZATION

1. Clean and dry all laboratory ware properly.
2. Cover open ends of the beaker, cylinder and other wide mouth containers with appropriate covering material, e.g. aluminium foil, brown paper, etc.
3. Keep surgical supplies, e.g. clamps, scalpel blade handles, forceps and scissors, etc. in stainless steel instrument trays. Wrap each article either individually or collectively by wrapping the tray as a whole.
4. Wrap softer articles such as surgeon towels, drapes and gowns, etc. individually.
5. For better security, wrap the articles by double wrapping into two sterilization sheets either sequentially [Fig. 5.1(A)] or simultaneously [Fig. 5.1(B)].

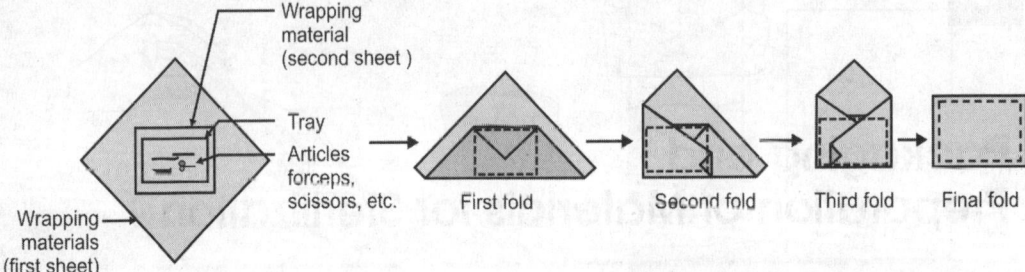

Fig. 5.1: (A) Sequential wrapping

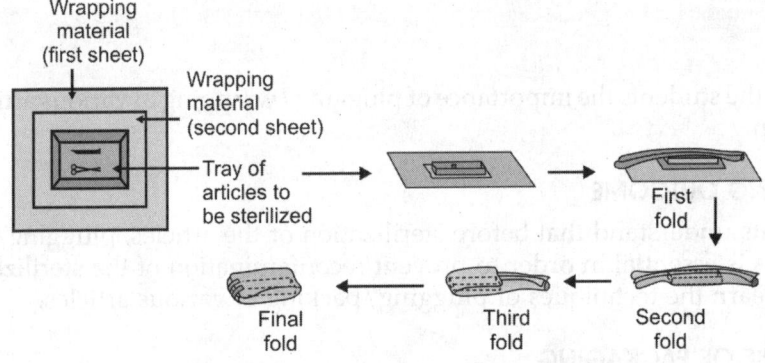

Fig. 5.1: (B) Simultaneous wrapping

5.5.1 Wrapping of Reusable Materials

Wrapping of all glass syringes: Separately place the plunger and barrel of properly washed all glass syringes on the same wrapping paper. Wrap them in the same paper along with the needle. Write the syringe capacity on the top of the packet.

Wrapping of petri dishes: Wrap clean petri dishes in small groups with heavy paper or place them in a petri dish can.

5.5.2 Plugging of Laboratory Test Tubes and Flasks

Carefully plug all test-tubes and flasks with non-absorbent cotton-wool.

1. For a test-tube or a small flask, tear a strip of cotton-wool some 10 cm long by 2 cm wide from the roll.
2. Turn in the ends neatly and roll the strip of wool lightly between the thumb and fingers of both hands to form a long cylinder (step 1).
3. Bend this at the centre and introduce the now rounded end into the open mouth of the tube or flask (step 2).
4. Now, whilst supporting the wool between the thumb and fingers of the right hand, rotate the test-tube and gradually screw the plug of wool into its mouth for a distance of about 2.5 cm leaving about the same length of wool projecting outside the tube (step 3).

The plug must be firm and fit the tube or flask, sufficiently tight, to bear the weight of the glass plus the amount of medium the vessel is intended to contain. It should be easily removed by a screwing motion when grasped between two fingers or the fingers and the palm of the hand (Fig. 5.2).

For a large flask, take a similar but larger strip of cotton wool; the method of making and inserting the plug is identical. Place an additional layer of gauge or cheese cloth under the cotton before inserting the plug into the mouth of the flask [Fig. 5.3 (b)].

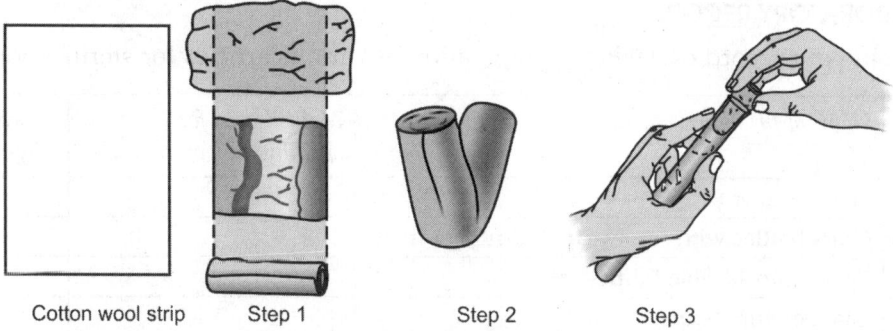

Cotton wool strip   Step 1   Step 2   Step 3

Fig. 5.2: Plugging of test tube (step 1)-Rolling of the cotton wool to make a cylinder, (step 2) folding of the cylinder, (step 3) insertion of the cotton wool plug

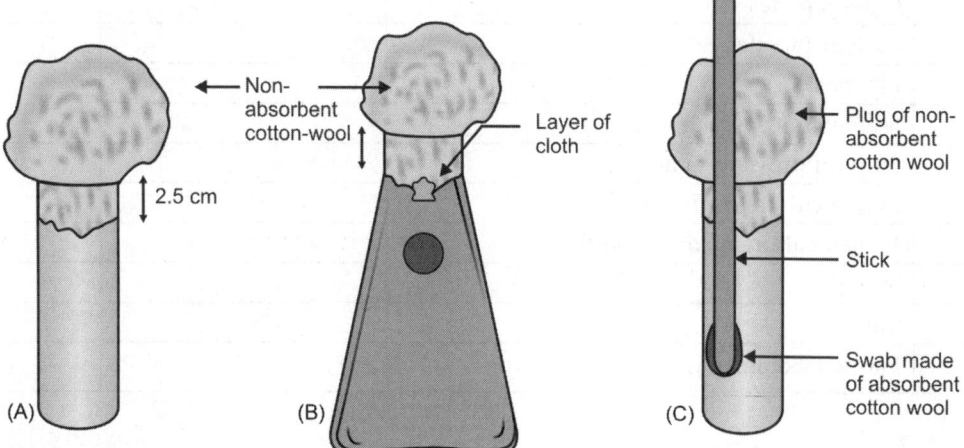

Fig. 5.3: (A) Plug on a test tube (B) Plug on an Erlenmeyer flask (C) Plug on a swab preparation

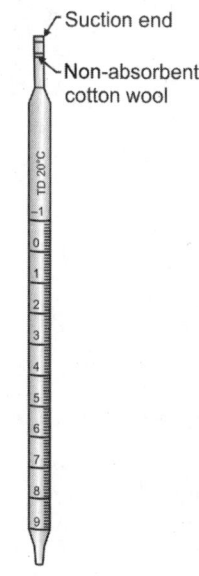

Fig. 5.4: Plugging of pipettes

If tubes are to be filled with a medium which is sterilized by autoclaving, do not plug until the medium is added. Both medium and tubes are thus sterilized with one autoclaving. If the tubes are to be filled with a sterile medium or if they are to be sterilized by the fractional method, plug the tubes/flasks before adding the medium.

Plugging of serological and bacteriological pipettes: Plug pipettes with about 10 mm of non-absorbent cotton-wool at the suction end and wrap individually in paper. Sterilize and store each variety in separate cylindrical copper cases approx 36 cm by 6 cm. with "pull-off" lid. Label the container with the capacity of the contained pipette (Fig. 5.4).

5.6 LABORATORY RECORD

Maintain your record of packing/preparation of various articles for sterilization

Date	Name of the material/articles	Method used for packing/preparation	Teacher's Signature
	Glass beaker		
	Glass bottles with screw cap and rubber liner		
	Glass autoclavable bottles		
	Glass culture bottles		
	Glass measuring cylinder		
	Glass centrifuge tube		
	Glass test tube		
	Glass pipettes		
	Pasteur pipettes		
	Pipettes		
	Scalpel, forceps, scissors, etc.		
	Surgical dressing materials		
	Liquid culture media in bottle		
	Molten culture media in bottle		
	Syringes		
	Cans		
	Plastic laboratory ware		

Equipment used for Sterilization

6.1 AIM

To educate students on principle of working, parts, proper operation and care of each equipment used for sterilization.

6.2 LEARNING OUTCOME

After this exercise, the students become familiar with the construction, working principle and operation of various sterilization equipment. They learn to operate each equipment taking proper care.

6.3 COMMON EQUIPMENT USED FOR STERILIZATION OF VARIOUS MATERIALS IN A CLINICAL LABORATORY

6.3.1 Hot Air Oven

6.3.1.1 Principle

Killing of organisms in the hot air oven is due to the oxidation of the cellular components of microorganisms by hot air.

6.3.1.2 Parts of a Simple Hot Air Oven (Fig. 6.1)

- Hot air oven is an electrically operated rectangular, double-walled metal box, mounted on a stand, heated from below and equipped with a fan to ensure uniform distribution of hot air inside the oven.
- One of the sides is hinged with a door.

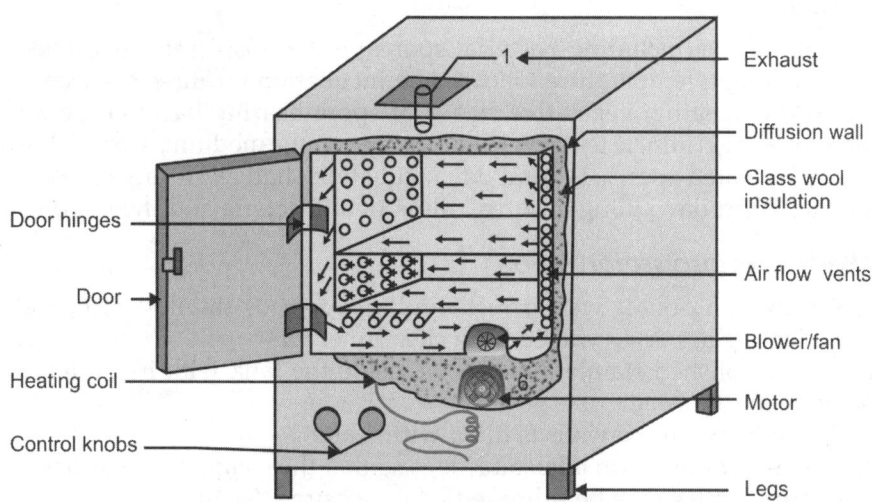

Fig. 6.1: Parts of a simple hot air oven

- The interior of the oven is provided with loose shelves upon which the articles to be sterilized are arranged.
- The top of the oven is provided with a cooling blower vent and air duct.
- The oven control switches may be located at the top or at the bottom depending on the manufacturer.
- There is a convection fan at the backside to distribute hot air evenly.

6.3.1.3 Operation of the Hot Air Oven

1. Arrange the materials (wrapped or unwrapped) to be sterilized loosely and evenly on the racks of the oven ensuring that the hot metal wall of the oven does not touch and char the cotton-wool plugs. While placing the materials, ensure that there is free flow of hot air inside the oven and uniform heating of the load.
2. Close the oven door and switch on the oven controlling the thermostat.
3. Monitor the internal temperature till it reaches 160°C **(heating up time).**
4. Wait for 2 hours allowing the temperature to remain at 160°C **(holding period)** (Table 6.1).
5. Switch off the hot air oven.
6. Allow the temperature of the interior, as recorded by the thermometer, to fall to 60°C in order to prevent cracking of the glass ware.
7. Open the door, remove the sterile articles and store them.

Table 6.1: Sterilization temperature and holding up time in a hot air oven

Article	Sterilization temperature	Holding up period
Wrapped items	170°C	60 min
	160°C	120 min
	150°C	150 min
	140°C	180 min
Unwrapped items	190°C	6 min
Dry heat (rapid flow) packaged item	190°C	12 min

6.3.2 Inspissator

6.3.2.1 Principle

Killing of organisms (including bacterial spores) in the inspissator is carried out by placing them at high temperature followed by incubation for three consecutive days. During first day heating, vegetative stages of spore bearing bacteria are killed. On incubation, spores germinate to the vegetative stage on the medium, second day heating kills these germinated spores. Second day incubation shall allow any left-over spores to germinate. Third day killing ensures killing of all bacteria and their spores.

6.3.2.2 Parts of an Inspissator (Fig. 6.2)

- Inspissator is a double-walled rectangular copper or stainless steel water tank with a loose glass or acrylic lid for a clear inner view.
- A shallow polished stainless tray rests inside the tank with its undersurface in contact with the water.
- The space between the walls is filled with water.
- The tray is supported on adjustable legs so that the coaguable material placed in the culture bottles may be solidified at any desired "slant,"
- It is heated from below by a heating element controlled by a thermo-regulator.

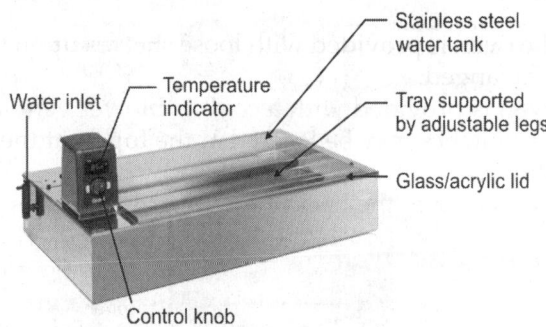

Fig. 6.2: Parts of an inspissator

6.3.2.3 *Operation of the Inspissator for Sterilization by Intermittent Heating Followed by Incubation*

1. Heat the water up to the desired temperature (usually 85°C for Lowenstein Jensen medium for tubercle bacilli).
2. Place the tubes/screw capped bottles with the medium containing serum/egg in the inspissator in a slanting position.
3. Keep them in the inspissator for 30 mins to 1 hour at desired temperature.
4. Remove the tubes/bottles from the inspissator.
5. Place the tubes/bottles in the incubator at 37°C for overnight.
6. Examine the tubes/bottles for growth, if any.
7. Place the tubes/bottles again in the inspissator for half an hour at the specific temperature.
8. Remove the tubes/bottles from the inspissator.
9. Place the tubes/bottles in the incubator at 37°C for overnight.
10. Place the tubes/bottles again in the inspissator for half an hour at the specific temperature.
11. Store the tubes/bottles in the refrigerator till further use.

6.3.3 Autoclave

6.3.3.1 Principle

Autoclaves destroy all forms of microorganisms by coagulation of their cell components by superheated and saturated steam under pressure. Autoclaves may be jacketed autoclave or non-jacketed autoclave, can be loaded vertically or horizontally or can be fully automated.

6.3.3.2 *Parts of a Simple Non-jacketed Autoclave* (Fig. 6.3)

A simple non-jacketed autoclave is like a pressure cooker having following parts:
- A leak proof cylindrical body made of a heavy duty metal.
- Heating element at the bottom.
- A lid fitted with an air tight gasket for closing the cylindrical structure, i.e. the body of autoclave.
- Screw clamps to close the body of the autoclave tightly with the lid and the gasket assembly.
- A pressure gauge and a safety valve placed on the top of the lid.

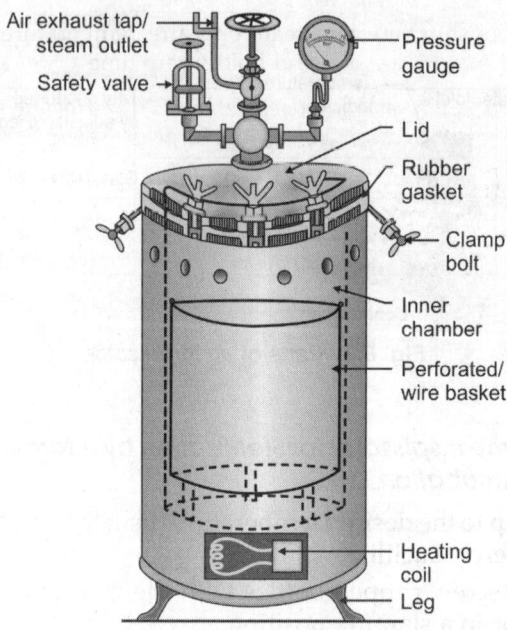

Fig. 6.3: Parts of a non-jacketed autoclave

Besides above essential parts, depending on the models, additional parts, e.g. handle, timer, pressure control knobs, lifting pedals for opening the autoclave, steam jackets, etc. may be present. Before use, you must get yourself acquainted with different parts of the particular autoclave you are handling and read the instructions carefully.

6.3.3.3 Operation of the Autoclave

1. Fill the autoclave with water up to the desired level.
2. Place properly packed materials in the wire basket.
3. Put the wire basket containing the materials for sterilization in the autoclave.
4. Ensure that the rubber gasket of the lid is in position.
5. Bolt the cover tightly onto the boiler by means of the clamp bolts.
6. Keep the air exhaust tap open and switch on the autoclave.
7. Ensure complete replacement of air by the steam as air and steam mixture results in a lower temperature at a particular pressure (Table 6.2). When steam starts coming out through the air discharge tap in a steady, continuous stream, close the outlet and let the steam pressure rise within the autoclave chamber.
8. Wait until the pressure gauge records the pressure of 15 psi./121°C or the desired pressure/temperature **(heating up time)**
9. Regulate the spring safety valve manually or automatically in such a manner that this pressure is just maintained, and leave it thus for twenty minutes **(holding time)**
10. Wait for 20 minutes (for 15 psi/121°C) (Table 6.2 shows the relationship between steam pressure, temperature of the superheated steam and holding up time depending on the sterilization load).
11. Switch off the autoclave and let it cool.
12. Wait till the pressure gauge has reached zero.
13. Slowly open the air and steam discharge taps.
14. Open the autoclave, take out the sterile materials.
15. Allow the materials to be cooled before they are handled.

Table 6. 2: Relationship between steam pressure, temperature of the superheated steam and holding up time

Steam pressure shown in the pressure gauge	Corresponding temperature of the steam with air discharge		Holding up period for sterilization with air discharge
	100%	50%	100%
5 psi	108.4°C	94°C	45 min–60 min
8 psi	112.6°C		30 min–45 min
10 psi	115.2°C	105°C	20 min–30 min
15 psi	121°C	112°C	15 min–20 min
20 psi	126°C	118°C	7 min–10 mins
30 psi	134.5°C	128°C	3 min (unwrapped items)
			8 min (lightly wrapped items)
			10 min (heavily wrapped items)

As seen from above table, steam temperature shall be considerably low if 100% of air is not discharged from the autoclave chamber.

6.3.4 Sterilization by Filtration

6.3.4.1 Principle

Filtration is the passage of a liquid or gas through a screen like material having very small pores to retain microorganisms. Membranes/HEPA filters retain microorganisms larger than their pore size on the surface of the filter when the liquid/gas passed through them.

Commonly used filters are:

6.3.4.2 Membrane Filters

Membrane filters or "membranes" are plastic films (mixed cellulose esters including cellulose nitrate and cellulose acetate, also known as nitrocellulose) having specific pore sizes to remove different size of microorganisms (Fig. 6.4)

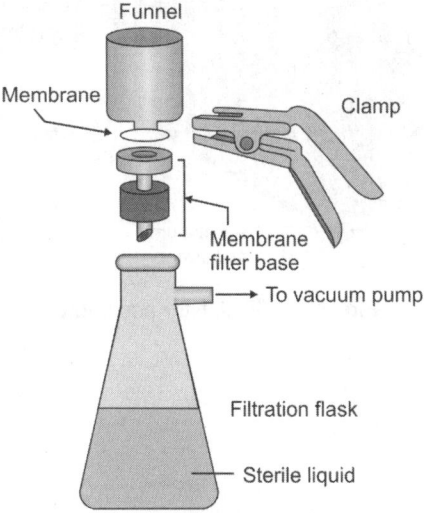

Funnel

Membrane

Clamp

Membrane filter base

To vacuum pump

Filtration flask

Sterile liquid

Fig. 6.4: Membrane filtration assembly

Membrane Filtration

Working principle membrane filtration is mostly carried out in flasks or in syringes for obtaining sterile liquid by creating vacuum or negative pressure in the receiving flask or in the syringe. As fluid passes through the filter, organisms are trapped in the pores of the membrane.

Parts of a Membrane Filtration Assembly

Parts of a membrane filtration assembly consist of:

- A heavy duty sterile flask with aside arm plugged with cotton wool.
- Tube connecting the side arm of the filtering flask with a vacuum pump.
- Funnel with the filter placed on the top of the flask (Fig. 6.4).

Procedure

1. Pour the unsterile liquid on the filter.
2. Turn on the vacuum pump connected through the side tube of the filtering flask.

The solution that drips into the receiving container is sterile. Microorganisms are trapped in the membrane.

6.3.4.3 High Efficiency Particulate Air filters (Fig. 6.5)

High efficiency particulate air (HEPA) filters are constructed from paper-like glass fibre or polymer sheets and are pleated many times to maximize the surface area within a small volume to enhance their effectiveness (Fig. 6.5).

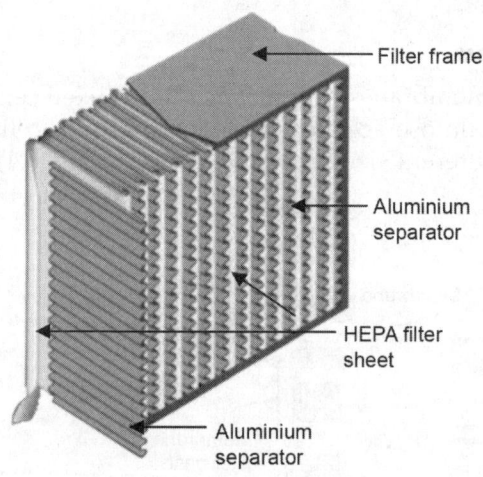

Filter frame

Aluminium separator

HEPA filter sheet

Aluminium separator

Fig. 6.5: HEPA filter assembly

6.4 LABORATORY RECORD

Familiarize yourself with the construction, operation and maintenance of each of the sterilizing equipment available in your laboratory. Maintain the record as under:

Date	Equipment operated	Precaution taken		Teacher's signature
		During operation	After operation	

Sterilization of Various Articles

7.1 AIM

To teach the students the differences amongst the terms sterilization, disinfection and antiseptic agents and selection of appropriate equipment/methods/materials for sterilizations of various articles.

7.2 LEARNING OUTCOME

After this exercise, the students learn the concepts of sterilization, disinfection and antisepsis. They can sterilize/disinfect different articles/areas using appropriate equipment/material and method.

7.3 STERILIZATION

Sterilization refers to any process that destroys or removes (by filtration) all forms of microbial life, including the spores that may be present on a surface, in a fluid, in a laboratory ware, in medication, or in a biological culture media.

Disinfection

Disinfection is the process of reducing microbial load/killing the microorganisms but may not be the bacterial spores. **Examples of disinfectants/bactericidal agents** are lysol, phenol, iodine, calcium hypochlorite, etc.

Antisepsis

Antisepsis is the process of prevention of further multiplication of bacteria. **Examples of antiseptic agents/bacteriostatic agents** are savlon, cetavelon, etc.

Sterilization can be achieved by

- **Physical methods** using heat, radiation, filter, etc.
- **Chemical methods** using **sterilant,** e.g. glutaraldehyde, hydrogen peroxide, etc. (liquid), ethylene oxide (gas).

7.3.1 Physical Agents for Sterilization

7.3.1 (a) Dry Heat

Dry heat kills organisms by oxidizing the essential cell constituents.

Dry heat is used in following forms/equipment depending on the articles to be sterilized:

- **Incinerator** (for destruction of morbid tissues, infected dead animals, spoiled dressings, sputum cups, etc. by heating to ashes)

- **Using hot air oven** for sterilizing dry materials such as glassware, syringes and needles, powders, gauze, bandages and other water immiscible substances like petroleum and oil. Heavy packets of fabric cannot be sterilized in hot air oven as penetration power of hot air is low.

- **Naked flame** for inoculating loop, inoculating needle **by heating them to redness,** forceps, rim of the tubes, etc. **by flaming for a short time** (Fig. 7.3). While sterilizing the inoculating loops by heating them to redness, the loop or needle must be held vertically in the non-luminous part of the Bunsen burner so as to cover maximum surface area. Temperature zone in the Bunsen burner flame is shown in Fig. 7.1 and correct procedure for sterilization by heating to redness shown at Fig. 7.2

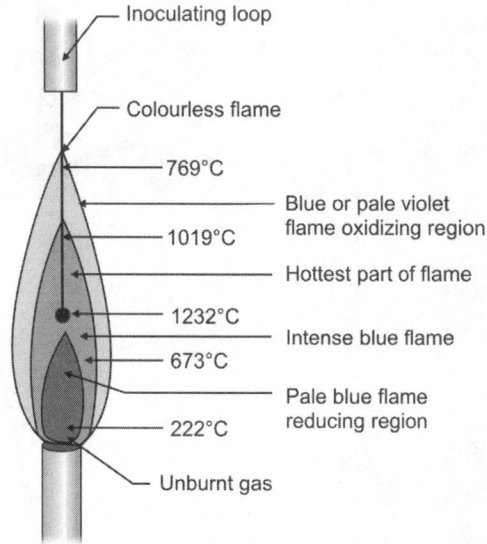

Fig. 7.1: Temperature zones in the Bunsen burner flame

A very short exposure to naked flame is employed for sterilizing the points of forceps, or other small instruments, cover-glasses, pipettes, rims of the test tubes, etc. Flaming of a screw capped bottle is shown in Fig. 7.3.

7.3.1 (b) Moist Heat: (Kills the Organisms by Coagulation of Cell Proteins)

Moist heat can be used in the following forms:

- **Water at 56°C or pasteurization** (mostly used for the removal of some pathogenic organisms in vegetative stage from milk. This method does not remove the thermophilic organisms and the spores of spore bearing organisms.

- **Water at 100°C** (for the sterilization of surgical instruments, rubber tubing, and stoppers, etc.). This method **does not ensure complete sterilization.**

- **Steam at 100°C (with intermittent overnight incubation at 37°C) for three consecutive days.** This method is called **tyndallization.** Spores are converted into vegetative stage during the period of incubation and the vegetative forms are destroyed during next exposure.

- **Superheated steam at 115°C or at 120°C** in the **autoclave** for the sterilization of **all articles except water immiscible articles, heat labile materials and heat**

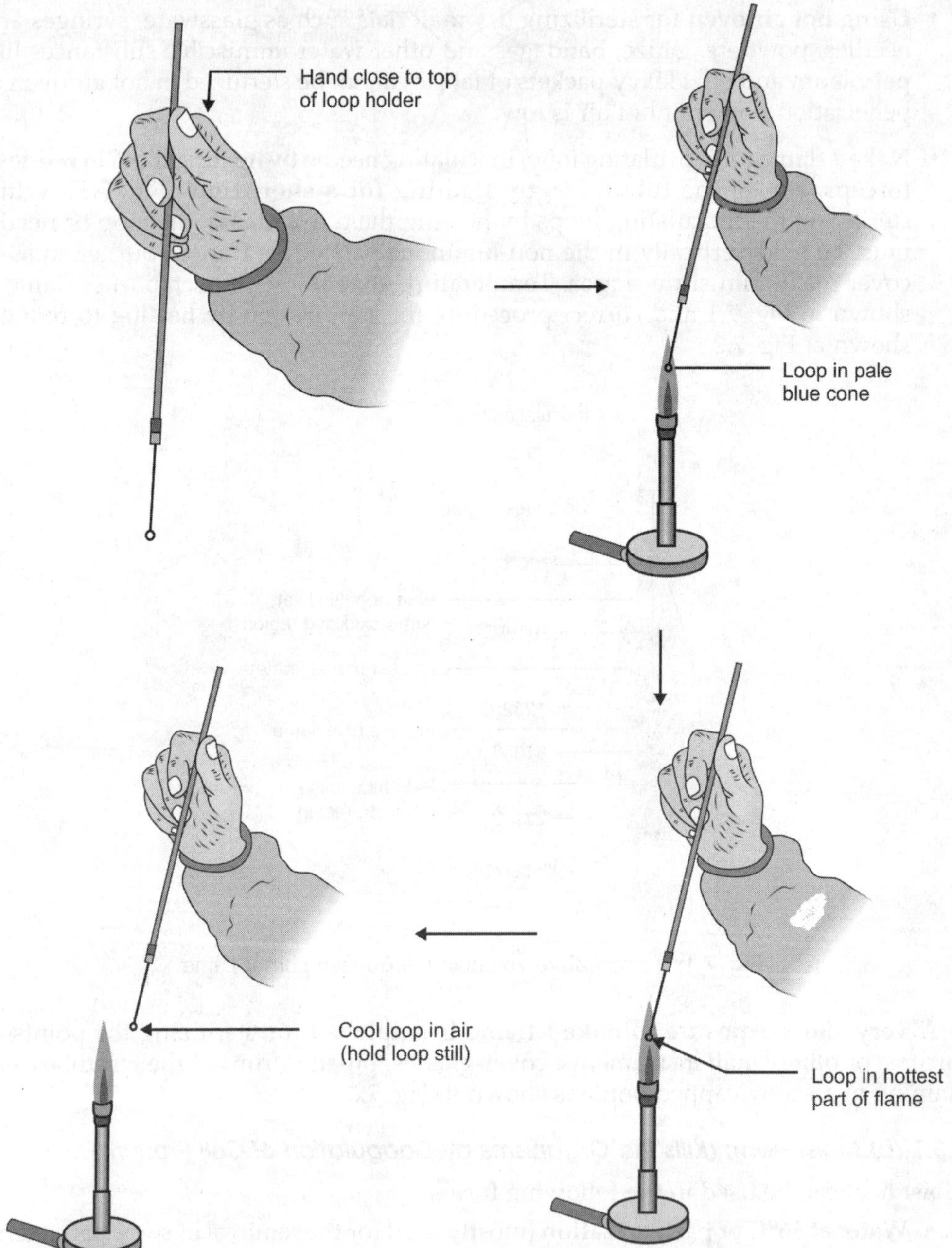

Hand close to top
of loop holder

Loop in pale
blue cone

Cool loop in air
(hold loop still)

Loop in hottest
part of flame

Fig. 7.2: Proper sterilization of an inoculating loop. Hold the loop handle by only the thumb and first two fingers and insert the loop vertically into the hottest part of the flame to sterilize maximum surface area. Cool loop by holding it in air.

coaguable materials. Steam under pressure is the most practical and dependable agent for sterilization as it provides higher temperature by rapid heating due to the latent heat released during condensation of steam and high penetration power of steam.

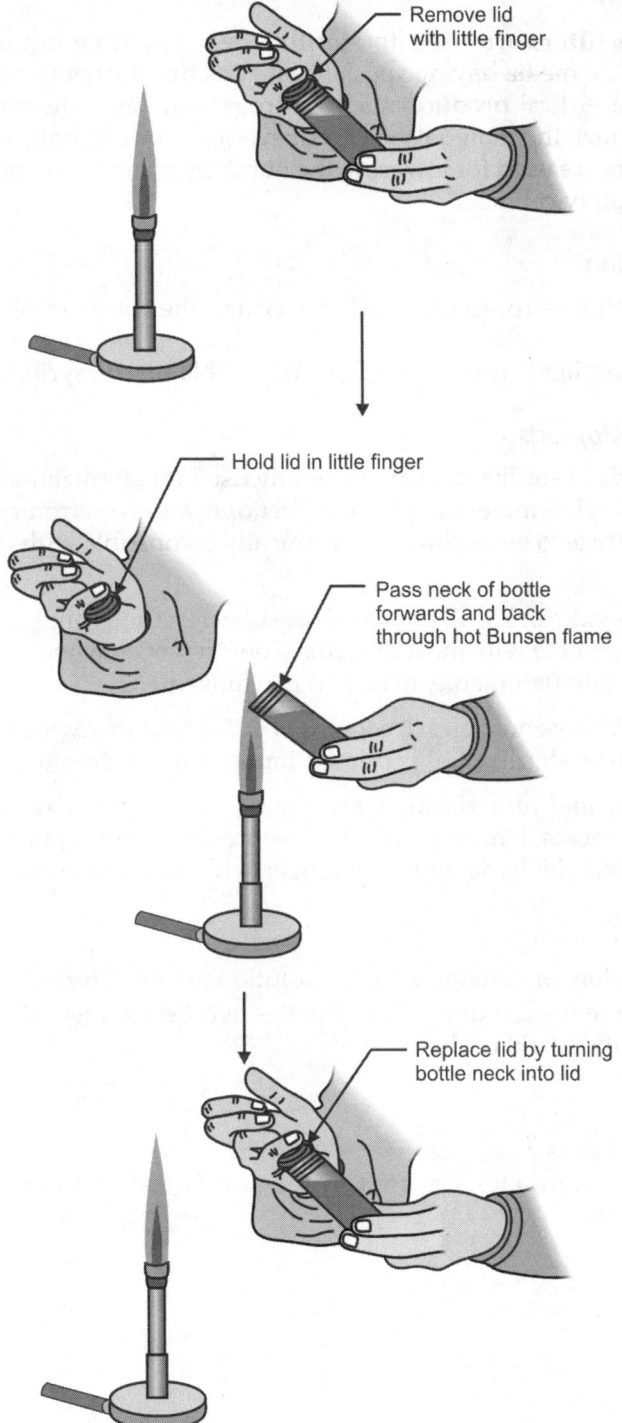

Fig. 7.3: Flaming of the screw capped bottle

7.3.1 (c) Filtration

- **Membrane filters** are used to sterilize heat sensitive liquid materials, e.g. bacteriological media having special heat-sensitive nutrients, enzymes, vaccines, and pharmaceutical products such as drugs, sera, and vitamins. They are also used to sterilize the materials such as beverages, intravenous solutions, etc.
- **HEPA filters** are used for lowering the numbers of air borne microbes and in the biological safety cabinets.

7.3.1 (d) Radiation

- **UV irradiation** is routinely used to sterilize the interiors of biological safety cabinets
- **Gamma radiation** is used to sterilize disposable plastic syringes.

7.3.2 Chemical Methods

Chemical methods of sterilization are generally used for sterilization of heat sensitive materials like biological materials, plastics, fiber optics and electronics items. One must ensure that the article to be sterilized is chemically compatible with the sterilant being used.

Ethylene oxide gas can kill all known viruses, bacteria and fungi, including bacterial spores and is compatible with most of medical devices, even when repeatedly applied. However, it is highly flammable, toxic and carcinogenic.

Chlorine bleach household bleach consists of 6.25% sodium hypochlorite. Depending on the material to be sterilized, it is diluted immediately before use.

Glutaraldehyde and formaldehyde solutions (also used as fixatives) are accepted liquid sterilizing agents. However, to kill all spores in a clear liquid, it may take up to 22 hours with glutaraldehyde and even longer with formaldehyde.

7.4 DISINFECTANT

Lysol, 2% solution, or carbolic acid, 5% solution are used for:
- Discarding the used slides, tubes, pipettes, etc. before they are sterilized.
- For wiping the workbench.

7.5 ANTISEPTICS

- Alcohol is used as a skin cleanser.
- Savlon, cetavalon, etc. are used in the wards for keeping instruments and thermometers.

7.6 LABORATORY RECORD

Record the methods and conditions followed by you for sterilization of following articles:

Date	Name of the material	Conditions for sterilization	Signature of teacher
	Glass beaker		
	Glass bottles with screw cap and rubber liner		
	Glass autoclavable bottles		
	Glass culture bottles		
	Glass cylinder		
	Centrifuge tube		
	Glass test tube		
	Glass pipettes		
	Pasteur pipettes		
	Pipettes		
	Scalpel, forceps, scissors, etc.		
	Surgical dressing materials		
	Liquid culture media in bottle		
	Molten culture media in bottle		
	Syringes		
	Pipette cans		
	Plastic laboratory ware		
	Urea solution		
	Inoculating loop		
	Serum		

8

Different Types of Microscopes: Handling and Care of Bright Field Microscope

8.1 AIM

To create awareness amongst the students on different types of microscopes along with a detailed study of compound (bright field) microscopes, their handling and care in the laboratory.

8.2 LEARNING OUTCOME

After this session, students become aware of the working principles of different types of microscopes, learn basic terms associated with microscopy, understand the movement of light path through various optical systems of a bright field microscope, learn the name and function of each part of a bright field microscope, can focus the objects with each objective lens and take proper care of the microscope while using the microscope and after completion of work.

Microscopes are the instruments used for viewing the magnified image of an object.

8.3 TYPES OF MICROSCOPES

Microscopes are broadly grouped as under:

Light microscope: Where light source is used for viewing the object.

Electron microscope: Where a beam of electrons are used in place of light and in-built magnets focus the electrons.

Scanning tunneling microscope (STM): Where instead of light or electron beam, a metal tip is held very close to the surface of the sample and electric current is measured as the tip passes over the atoms of the surface.

8.3.1 Light Microscopes are Further Divided as under

8.3.1.1 Bright Field Microscope

This is the most commonly used microscope. This uses a visible light source, either sunlight or electric bulb, for seeing both dry preparation and wet preparation of an object. Path of light through a bright field microscope is shown in Fig. 8.1

8.3.1.2 Dark Field Microscope

This type of light microscope uses a modified condenser. The object is seen as a colorless body against a dark background. This microscope can be used to see the organisms in living stage. Path of light is shown in Fig. 8.2.

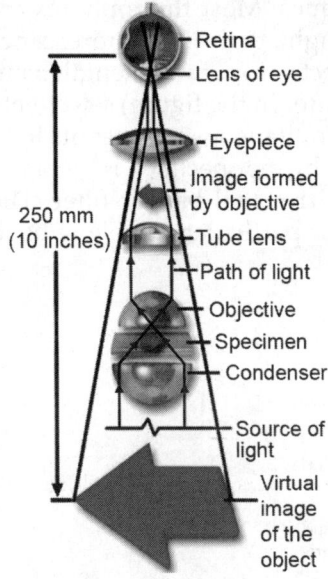

Fig. 8.1: Path of light in a bright field microscope

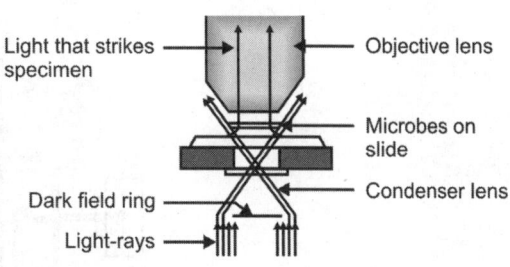

Fig. 8.2: Path of light in dark field microscope

8.3.1.3 Phase Contrast Microscope

This microscope uses a special condenser that enhances the small difference in the refractive index and density between the living cells and the fluid in which they are suspended. Path of light is shown in Fig. 8.3.

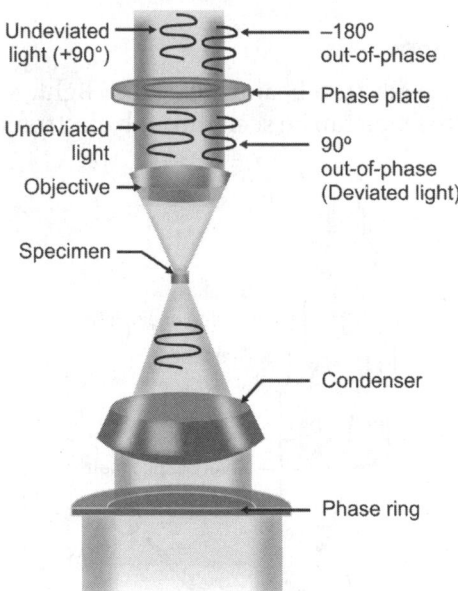

Fig. 8.3: Light path in a phase contrast microscope

8.3.1.4 Fluorescence Microscope

Fluorescence microscopes use light sources that can emit both ultraviolet and visible light spectrum. Depending on the nature of fluorescein conjugated reagents used, mercury arc lamp, xenon lamps, laser, LED, etc. are used as light sources. Lasers are used for more complex fluorescence microscopy techniques. Most fluorophores are excited by ultraviolet, blue, and green wavelengths. Light path in a fluorescence microscope is explained in Fig. 8.4, the excitation filter selects proper wavelength band for excitation. The dichromatic mirror (dichroic beam splitter in the figure) selectively reflects light with a particular range of wavelength and simultaneously transmits light of longer and shorter wavelengths. Fluorescence emission by the specimen is gathered by the objective and passes through the dichromatic mirror and barrier filter. The barrier filter is specifically designed to allow only light of particular wavelengths to reach the microscope eyepieces and/or detector.

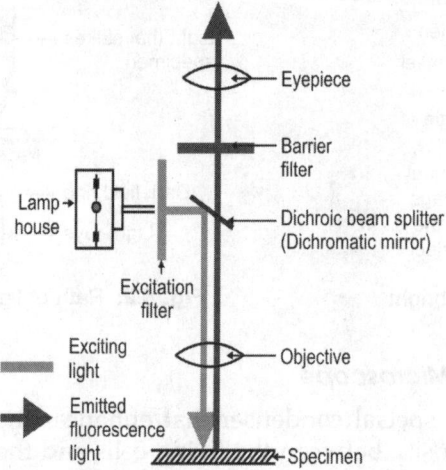

Fig. 8.4: Light path in a fluorescence microscope

8.3.2 Electron Microscopes

Electron microscopes use electron beams instead of light. Minute objects that are not visible under light microscope can be seen through electron microscope. Electron path is shown in Fig. 8.5.

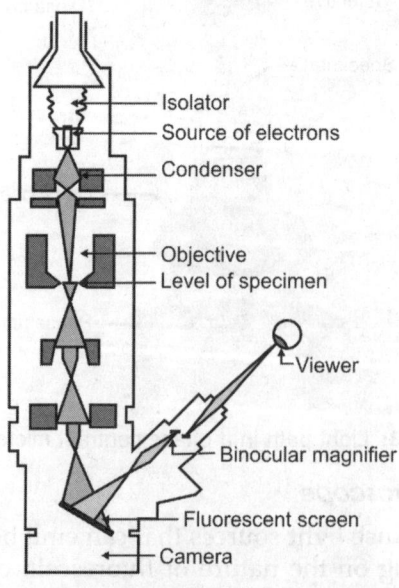

Fig. 8.5: Path of electrons in an electron microscope

Relative sizes of microorganisms and their visibility under light microscope and electron microscope are shown in Fig. 8.6

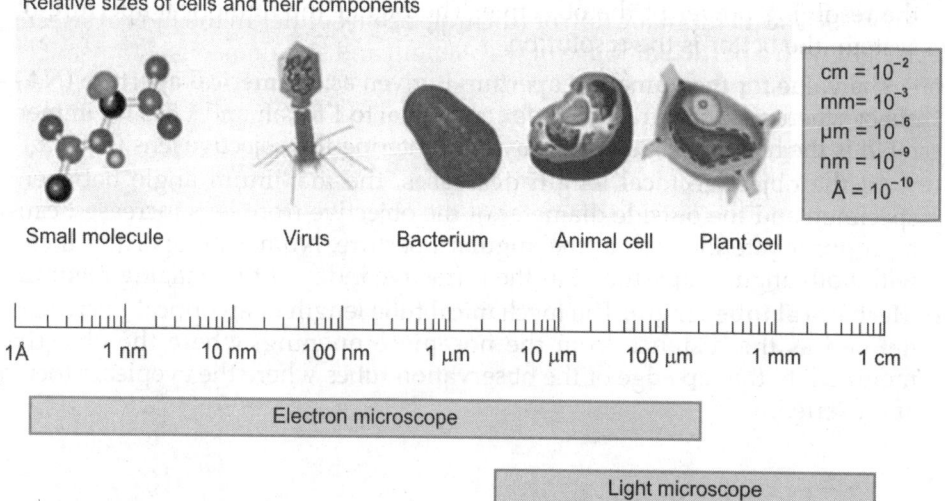

Fig. 8.6: Relative sizes of microorganisms and their visibility under different microscopes

8.3.2.1 Bright Field Microscopy

Principle: Bright field microscopes use ordinary light source to magnify a small object or to view the finer details of a large object. Compound microscope uses two sets of lenses—the objective lens that makes an enlarged image of the object and the ocular lens or eyepiece that further magnifies that image (Fig. 8.1). Total magnification is expressed as the power of the objective lens multiplied by the power of the eyepiece lens.

Terms used in bright field microscopy

a. **Total magnification is the** magnification by the objective × magnification by the eyepiece. With 10X eyepiece, when 10X, 40X and 100X objectives are used, the total magnification of the object is 100 times, 400 times and 1000 times respectively.

b. **Working distance:** This is the distance between the objective and the object, (approximately 5 mm for 10X, 0.35 mm for 40X and 0.1 mm for 100X objective) (Fig. 8.7).

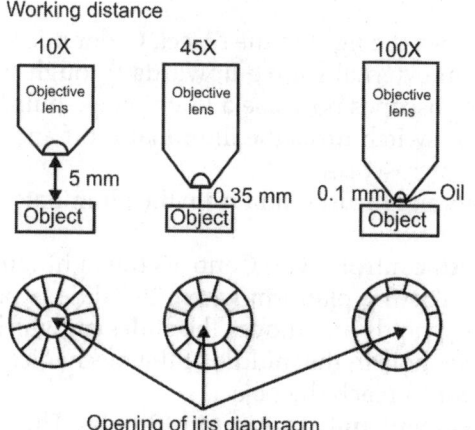

Fig. 8.7: Approximate working distance and front lens diameter of the 10X, 40X and 100X) objectives and opening of the iris diaphragm for each objective

c. **Resolution:** Resolution of a microscope is the smallest distance between two points on a specimen that can be labeled as separate entities.

d. **Numerical aperture:** The numerical aperture of a microscope objective determines the resolving power of the objective. The higher the numerical aperture of the system, the better is the resolution.

The value for the numerical aperture is given as: **Numerical aperture (NA)** = n **sin α,** where n is the refractive index and equal to 1 for air and 1.515 for immersion oil. α is the half angle subtended by rays entering the objective lens (Fig. 8.8).

As the objective focal length decreases, the maximum angle between the specimen and the outside diameter of the objective front lens increases, causing a proportionate increase in the angular aperture. Numerical aperture increases with both angular aperture and the refractive index of the imaging medium.

e. **Mechanical tube length:** The mechanical tube length of an optical microscope is defined as the distance from the nosepiece opening, where the objective is mounted, to the top edge of the observation tubes where the eyepieces (oculars) are inserted.

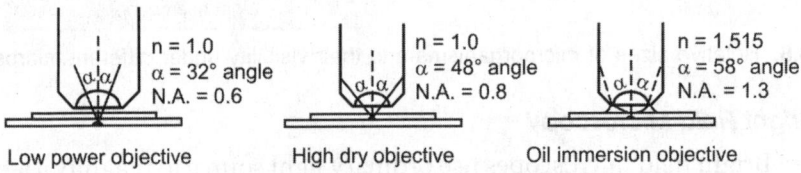

n = 1.0 α = 32° angle N.A. = 0.6	n = 1.0 α = 48° angle N.A. = 0.8	n = 1.515 α = 58° angle N.A. = 1.3
Low power objective	High dry objective	Oil immersion objective

n refractive index, NA Numerical aperture
α is the half angle subtended by rays entering the objective lens

Fig. 8.8: Numerical aperture for various objectives

Parts of a Compound Microscope (Fig. 8.9)

Each compound microscope has the structural parts (consisting of the body tube, arm, stage, base, etc.) and the optical parts (comprising of light source, lenses, condenser, diaphragm, etc.). Optical parts are attached to the structural part.

Names and function of individual parts are given as under:

- **Base:** The base supports the microscope and the light source is located on the base.
- **Light source:** Supplies the light to the object. Older microscopes used mirrors to reflect light from an external source upwards through the bottom of the stage; however, most microscopes now use a low-voltage bulb.
- **On/off switch:** This switch turns the illuminator off and on. This is also located on the base of the microscope.
- **Condenser:** Gathers and focuses light from the illuminator/mirror onto the object being viewed.
- **Iris diaphragm with control lever:** Controls the light falling on the object.
- **Mechanical stage:** The flat platform where the slide is placed. With the help of stage clips, the stage holds and moves the slides on which the object is placed.
- **Aperture:** This is the hole in the middle of the mechanical stage that allows light from the illuminator to reach the object.
- **Stage height adjustment and stage control knobs:** These knobs move the stage left and right or up and down.
- **Stage clips:** Metal clips on the stage that hold the slide in place.

- **Objective lenses:** Objective lenses are the lenses closest to the object. There may be three, four, or five objective lenses that produces magnified image of the object. These lenses range in power from 4X to 100X.
- **Revolving nosepiece:** The rotating structure that houses the objective lenses and brings the desired objective lens into position above the object.
- **Coarse adjustment:** Brings the object into general focus.
- **Fine adjustment:** Fine tunes the focus and facilitates detailed examination of the specimen.
- **Arm:** The arm connects the body tube to the base of the microscope.
- **Body tube:** The body tube connects the eyepiece to the objective lenses.
- **Diopter adjustment:** Useful as a means to change focus on one eyepiece so as to correct for any difference in vision between the two eyes of the viewer.
- **Eyepiece:** The lens through which the viewer looks to see the specimen. The eyepiece usually contains 10X or 15X power lens.

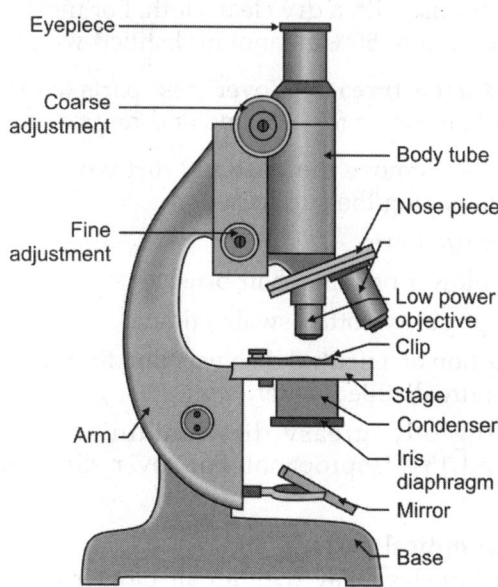

Fig. 8.9: Parts of an optical microscope

Operation of the Microscope

1. Place the microscope on a solid table so that it does not vibrate.
2. Keep the stage on a horizontal position so that the immersion oil or other liquids do not run off the slide .
3. If the microscope is provided with a mirror, adjust the mirror in respect to the source of light. For a distant source of light, concave mirror will yield better illumination. For a closely placed light source, use the plain side of the mirror. If the microscope has a built- in illuminator, switch it on.
4. Use 10X objectives for adjusting the illumination.
5. Focus the condenser and adjust the iris diaphragm and condenser so that ¾ of the lens is filled with light. This illumination may vary with different objects.
6. Place the slide on the stage with the desired viewing area of the object placed above the aperture. Use cover glass whenever required.

7. Bring 10X objectives near its working distance (approx 5 mm) above the area of the object to be seen. Gently move it up and down with the coarse focusing knob until the image comes in view. Focus it sharply with the fine adjustment knob.

8. Turn the mirror/adjust the illuminator until the image is at its brightest.

9. Examine the specimen by moving the slide with the help of the mechanical stage.

10. For 40X objectives, place the desired area of the object at the centre of field of vision of the 10X objective. Place the high power objective on the slide and focus the object with fine adjustment. Adjust the iris for the particular object.

11. For 100X objective, open the iris completely, place a drop of immersion oil on the object and examine the specimen taking extreme care in moving the 100X objective.

Cleaning the Microscope

Metallic surfaces: Wipe off dust with a dry clean cloth. For more persistent dirt, use a mild neutral detergent solution or 50% ethanol in distilled water.

Mechanical guides and screw threads: Cover these parts with a thin film of grease. Protect from solvents. Call an expert for cleaning and re-greasing of these parts.

Optical parts: Completely remove the dust and dirt without leaving any residue of the cleaning agent or damaging the surfaces.

Cleaning materials required are:

- Dust blower or bulb blower or camel hair brush.
- Soft lens tissue or high purity cotton swabs/tissue.
- Freshly prepared solution of a neutral dish washing liquid (5 to 10 drops in 10 ml of distilled water or pure distilled water.
- Solvent for removing oily/greasy dirt containing 85% petroleum ether (analytically pure) and 15% isopropanol. For cover slips, pure acetone may be used.

Cleaning procedure for optical parts:

1. Blow all loose dust particles away with an air blower with a rubber bulb or a clean camel hair brush.
2. Remove all water soluble dirt with a soft cotton or tissue soaked in distilled water.
3. For persistent dirt, use dilute washing liquid.
4. Remove oily residue first with the dilute washing liquid. Then, if required, with the solvent.
5. Remove greasy residue with the petroleum ether- isopropanol mixture using a spiral motion from centre to the rim of the optical surface with very little direct force on the optical surface.
6. Discard the lens paper/tissue paper after a single use.

Clean all optical parts of the microscope every time before and after use: Never expose the lacquered part of the microscope to the lens cleaning solution as this will dissolve the lacquer.

Care of the Microscope

1. Keep the microscope free from dust.
2. Use both hands to grasp the microscope with one hand holding the arm and the other hand holding the bottom of the base.
3. Never jar or tip over the microscope.
4. Always clean the optical parts of the microscope with a lens paper/lint less tissue paper soaked in a lens cleaner. Never use ordinary paper or any rough fabric to clean the optical parts. This will damage the lens/optical parts.
5. Periodically lubricate the mechanical parts with a good machine oil.
6. Never allow violent contact of the object lens with the slide. It may ruin the objective.
7. Never allow immersion oil to dry on the oil immersion objective. Clean the objective after each use.
8. Take precaution against fungal growth by keeping a desiccant in the microscope box or lighting an electric bulb inside the microscope box.

Checklist for Care of Microscope

Action required before and after use	Daily/after each use	Weekly when not in use	Annually
Remove slide	✓		
Clean objectives with lens paper	✓	✓	
Adjust optic system	✓		
Clean optic system externally	✓	✓	
Clean mechanical parts externally	✓	✓	
Cover with dust cover	✓	✓	
Overhauling by professionals			✓

8.3.2.2 Laboratory Record

Record your compliance with following activities:

Date	Compliance with following activities						Teacher's signature
	Removed slide	Cleaned objectives with lens paper	Adjusted optic system	Cleaned optic system externally	Cleaned mechanical parts externally	Covered with dust cover	

Examination of Morphology of Microorganisms under Bright Field Microscope

9.1 AIM

To educate the students about different types of microorganisms that are visible under ordinary microscopes and their morphological features.

9.2 LEARNING OUTCOME

After completing this session, students are able to differentiate between bacteria, fungi and protozoa under the microscope. They can make general classification of the bacteria based on their shape and arrangement.

9.3 GENERAL MORPHOLOGY OF BACTERIA

Bacteria are unicellular organisms having characteristics cellular structure.

Morphologically, bacteria possess three main shapes: spherical, cylindrical (rod shaped) or spiral and are known as coccus (pleural cocci), bacillus (pleural bacilli) and spirillum (pleural spirilla) respectively (Fig. 9.1).

Coccus: Coccus (pleural cocci) may have spherical, ellipsoidal, bean shape or lanceolate shape. Based on their arrangement, cocci are subdivided into six groups:

1. Micrococci: arranged singly or irregularly.
2. Diplococci: remain in pairs.
3. Streptococci: arranged in chains of different lengths.
4. Staphylococci: arranged in groups resembling clusters of grapes.
5. Tetracocci: remains in group of 4 cocci.
6. Sarcinae: resembles packets of 8, 16 or more cells.

Bacilli (Rod like bacteria) are subdivided into:

1. Bacterium that are non-sporing rods.
2. Bacillus that are aerobic spore bearing rods.
3. *Clostridium* that are anaerobic spore bearing rods.
4. Actinomycetes that forms branching filaments.
5. Fusiforms that are enlarged rod with tapering ends.

Spiral shaped bacteria are sub-classified as:

1. Vibrio: which looks like a comma.
2. Spirillum: which are coiled form of bacteria having twists with one or more turns.
3. Spirochete: these are shaped like a cork screw.

Shape	Name	Classification based on arrangement	Other features
Spherical	Coccus (pleural cocci)	• Diplococci 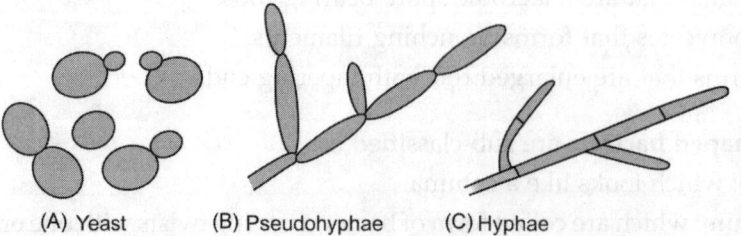 • Tetrad • Sarcinae • *Streptococcus* • *Staphylococcus* • *Micrococcus*	Coffee bean shaped diplococci or plano convex (Neisseria)
Rod like	Bacillus	• Diplobacilli • Streptobacilli • Bacilli arranged in palisades	• Coccobacilli • Aerobic and anaerobic spore bearers • Fusiform • Filamentous • With granules Budding and appendaged bacteria — Hypha / Stalk
Curved	Vibrio/ spirillum/ spirochetes/ helicobacteria	• Vibrio • Helical • Spiral • Spirochetes	

Fig. 9.1: Morphology and arrangement of bacteria

9.4 GENERAL MORPHOLOGY OF FUNGUS (PLEURAL FUNGI)

Fungi are unicellular or multicellular organisms bigger in size than that of bacteria. They multiply by budding (yeast form) or by producing hyphae with spores that vary in size, shape and structure (Fig. 9.2).

(A) Yeast   (B) Pseudohyphae   (C) Hyphae

Fig. 9.2: Morphology of fungi (A) yeast form, (B and C) mold forms

9.5 GENERAL MORPHOLOGY OF PROTOZOA

Protozoa are non-photosynthetic unicellular organisms with protoplasm clearly differentiated into nucleus and cytoplasm. Main divisions of protozoa includes:

- Ameba: That moves by extending pseudopodia (Fig. 9.3)
- Sporozoa: All are intracellular parasites (Fig. 9.4)
- Flagellates: Which moves by beating one or more flagella (Fig. 9.5)
- Ciliates: Move with the help of many cilia (Fig. 9.6)

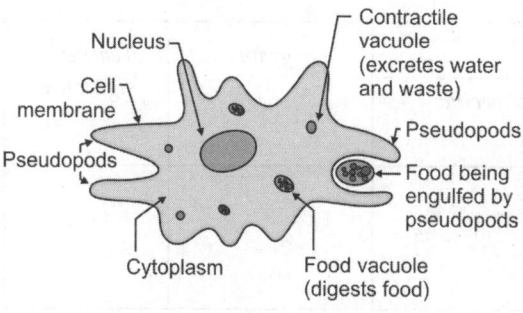

Fig. 9.3: Protozoa (ameba)

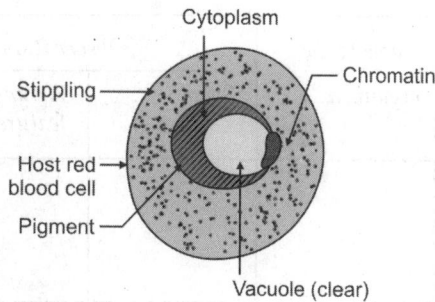

Fig. 9.4: Protozoa (sporozoa) malaria parasite inside the red blood cell

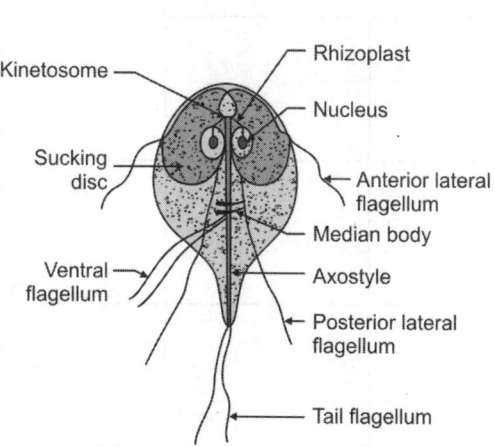

Fig. 9.5: Protozoa: flagellate (Giardia)

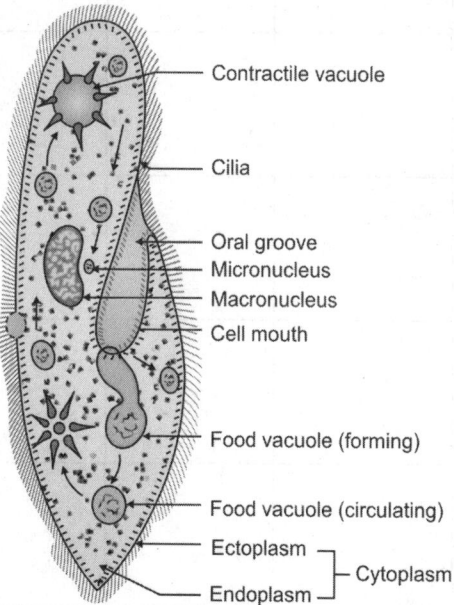

Fig. 9.6: Protozoa: ciliate (Paramecium)

9.6 EXAMINATION OF MICROORGANISMS UNDER THE MICROSCOPE

9.6.1 Materials Required

- Microscope with oil immersion objective.
- Preserved slides of known organisms.

9.6.2 Procedure

1. Place the slide on the stage of the microscope.
2. Focus the specific area first with 10X objective, then with 40X and finally with 100X objective after applying a drop of oil (especially in case of bacteria).
3. Report your observation and draw diagrams of the organisms seen.

9.7 LABORATORY RECORD

Record your observation as under:

Date

Name of the organism	Observation		Diagram	Teacher's signature
	Shape	*Arrangement/specific feature, if any*		

Simple Staining

10.1 AIM

To teach the students the technique of preparing bacterial film, staining them with a single dye and to examine the preparation for studying the morphology of bacteria.

10.2 LEARNING OUTCOME

After completing the exercise, students can make bacterial film/smear on a slide, stain them with a single dye (methylene blue) and observe their morphology under the microscope.

10.3 PRINCIPLE

Bacterial protoplasm is acidic in nature. Therefore, they can be stained with basic dyes, i.e. dyes having their colour in the cationic part, e.g. methylene blue (MB) has the structure MB^+, Cl^-. Methylene blue colour is present at the cationic part. MB^+ combines with the bacterial cell to give it a blue colour.

10.4 MATERIALS REQUIRED

- 24 hours broth culture and agar culture of different bacteria
- Inoculating loop (in case of broth culture) and inoculating needle (in case of growth on agar plate)
- Clean slides
- Sterile saline
- 0.5% methylene blue solution
- Immersion oil

10.5 PREPARATION OF THE STAINING SOLUTION

0.5% methylene blue staining solutions

- Take 0.5 gm of methylene blue powder and dissolve in 100 ml distilled water.

10.6 PREPARATION OF THE BACTERIAL SMEAR

10.6.1 From Bacterial Colony

1. Take a clean slide. Heat one side to remove any grease.
2. Sterilize the inoculating loop by holding it in Bunsen burner flame till it becomes red.
3. Wait a little to cool the loop by holding it near the flame itself.
4. Take one loopful of sterile saline with aseptic precaution and place it at the centre of the slide.

5. Sterilize the loop once again and place it in the rack.

6. Sterilize the inoculating needle in the flame by holding it vertically in the flame and heating it to redness. Cool it while holding the needle near the flame.

7. Pick up a minute growth from the colony with aseptic precaution and emulsify it in the saline at the centre of the slide to make a smear of about 2 cm × 1 cm size.

8. Sterilize the needle again and keep it in the needle stand.

9. Allow the smear to dry.

10. Quickly pass the slide five to six times through the flame to fix the smear so that it does not get washed off during subsequent staining steps and also to kill the cells so that they allow the stain to enter inside.

11. Mark the smear on the other side of the slide and write the name of the bacteria.

10.6.2 From Broth Culture

1. Take the clean slide and heat one side to make it grease free.

2. Sterilize the inoculating loop by holding it vertically in the flame till it is red hot. Cool it near the flame.

3. Aseptically take one loopful of broth culture with the sterile inoculating loop and place it on the centre of the slide. Emulsify to make a smear of about 2 cm × 1 cm.

4. Sterilize the inoculating loop and place it in its stand.

5. Dry the smear, fix it and mark it on the other side.

10.6.3 Staining of the Smear

1. Cover the smear with the methylene blue staining solution

2. Keep for 30 seconds.

3. Drain off the staining solution.

4. Wash with tap water.

5. Drain dry and then air dry.

6. Observe under oil immersion objective.

Flow chart 10.1: Simple staining

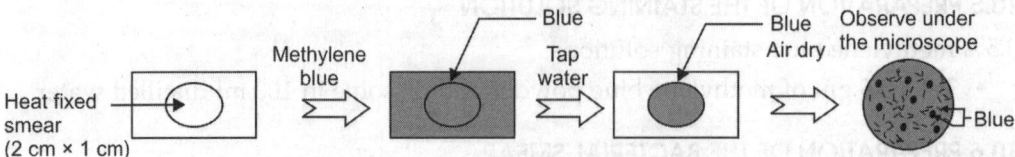

10.7 LABORATORY RECORD

1. Prepare smears from different bacterial cultures and stain them by simple staining.

2. Add one drop of immersion oil on the stained smear.

3. Place the slide on the microscope stage and examine under 100× (oil immersion objective).

4. Record your finding completing following table.

Date

Name of the organism	Staining solution used	Observation		Teacher's signature
		Colour	*Shape, arrangement and inclusions, if any.*	

Demonstration of
Bacterial Motility by Hanging Drop Method

11.1 AIM

To teach the students the importance of detection of bacterial motility under the microscope and the method of examination of true motility.

11.2 LEARNING OUTCOME

After this exercise, the students are able to detect bacterial motility under the microscope and can differentiate between true motility (vital movement) and Brownian movement.

11.3 PURPOSE

Hanging drop experiment helps in the preliminary identification of bacteria based on their motility.

11.4 PRINCIPLE

True motility or vital movement of bacterial cell is characterized by a wriggling, tumbling or darting movement of a bacterial cell by which the organism changes its location from one place to another. This movement is mostly due to the presence of the organ of locomotion, i.e. flagella (Fig. 11.1) Other kind of movement seen in a liquid medium is the Brownian movement wherein the bacteria remain in the same place with back and forth movement due to molecular bombardment with the liquid molecules (Fig. 11.3).

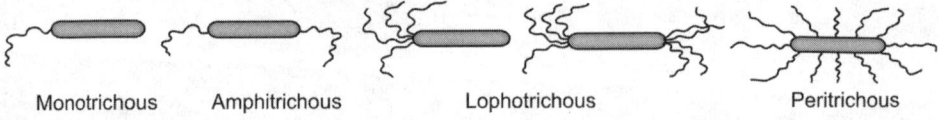

| Monotrichous | Amphitrichous | Lophotrichous | Peritrichous |

Fig. 11.1: Bacterial flagella and nomenclature of flagella based on the position and number of flagella

11.5 MATERIALS REQUIRED

- 2–4 hours broth culture of bacteria
- Slides and cover slips or cavity slides
- Plasticin/modeling clay
- Inoculating loop

11.6 PROCEDURE

1. Using plasticin or modeling clay, make a ring with an approximate inner diameter of 1 cm.
2. Place it at the centre of a clean slide.

3. Aseptically place a drop of the bacterial culture in the centre of a clean cover slip taking care that the drop does not spread.
4. Invert the slide with plasticin ring and carefully place it on the cover slip to bring the droplet at the centre of the plasticin ring.
5. Re-invert the slide with the adhering cover slip and place it on the stage of the microscope so that the cover slip faces the objective with the droplet "hanging" from the inner side of the cover slip (Fig. 11.2).

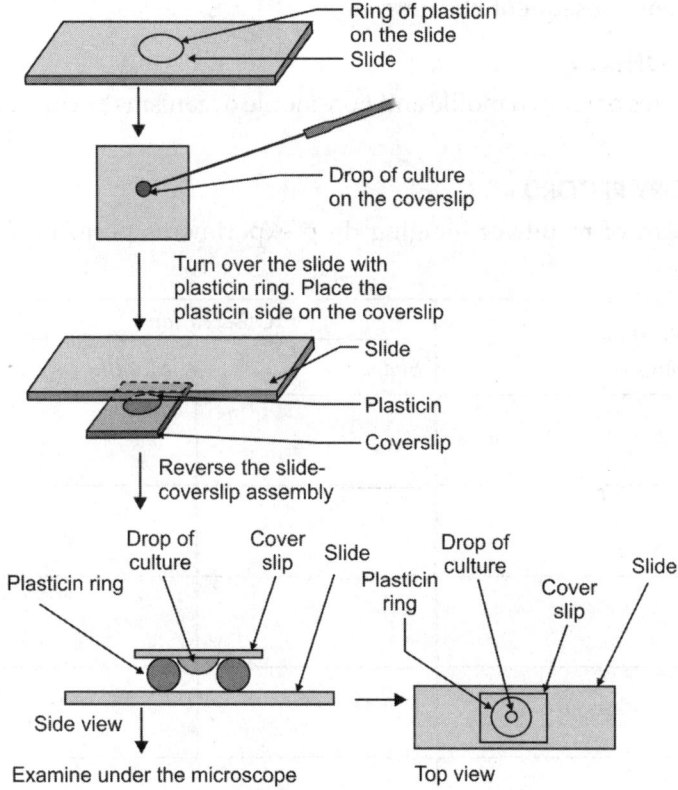

Fig. 11.2: Hanging drop preparation with a plasticin ring and examination of bacterial motility

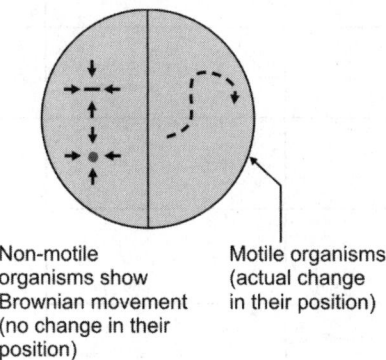

Fig. 11.3: Motile and non-motile bacteria under the microscope

6. Reduce the light by adjusting the diaphragm and the condenser.
7. First focus the edge of the drop with a 10× objective and bring it at the centre of the field of vision.
8. Now focus the edge with the high dry objective.
9. Once the edge is focused, move the slide carefully to view various parts of the drop for examining the motility of bacteria. Check for true motility and Brownian movement (Fig. 11.3).
10. If available, you may use a cavity slide for placing the drop of culture and examine the drop.
11. After examination, discard the slides and cover slips in disinfectant solution before their subsequent cleaning.

11.7 QUALITY CONTROL

Take broth cultures of known motile and non-motile organisms as controls and examine their motility.

11.8 LABORATORY RECORD

Maintain a record of results of hanging drop experiments performed by you in the following table:

Date	Name of the organism	Observation		Teacher's signature
		Shape	Motility	

Gram Staining

12.1 AIM

To educate the students about the importance of Gramstaining in a clinical microbiology laboratory and the technique of Gram staining with necessary quality control.

12.2 LEARNING OUTCOME

After this exercise, the students understand the basic principle of Gram staining and the importance of gram staining in a microbiology laboratory. They also learn to carry out Gram staining independently.

12.3 PURPOSE

Purpose of Gram staining: To do preliminary identification of the organisms based on their Gram character.

12.4 PRINCIPLE

Gram staining divides the microorganism into two groups on the basis of their ability to retain the primary stain. The group that retains the primary stain is called Gram-positive. The other group that cannot retain the primary colour on washing with alcohol are termed Gram-negative organisms. Most important structural differences in the cell walls of these two groups are: **Gram-positive organisms have thick (3 to 80 nm) peptidoglycan layer and Gram-negative organisms have thin peptidoglycan layer (5–10 nm) overlaid by an outer membrane of lipopolysaccharide–lipoproteins** (Fig. 12.1).

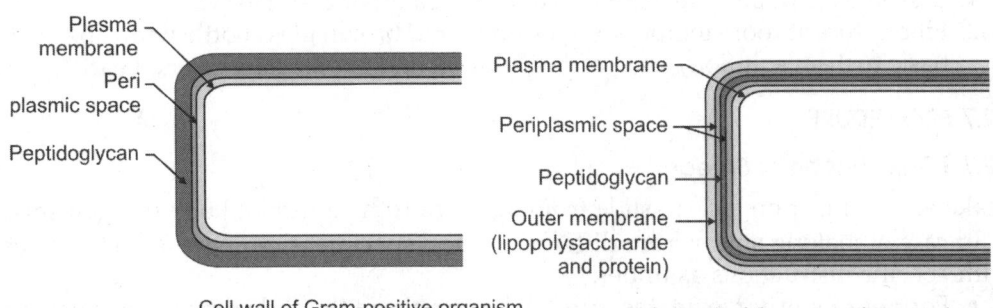

Fig. 12.1: Schematic diagram of the differences in the cell walls of Gram-positive and Gram-negative bacteria

12.5 MATERIALS REQUIRED

- Clean slides.
- Inoculating loop.
- Known bacterial culture or specimens of body fluid/material.
- Permanent marker or glass marker pen/pencil.
- Primary stain: methyl violet or crystal violet or gentian violet.
- Mordant: Gram's iodine or Lugol's iodine.
- Decolouriser: acetone-alcohol or acetone.
- Counter stain: safranin or basic fuchsin.
- Distilled water

12.6 PREPARATION OF THE REAGENTS

Primary stain: methyl violet or crystal violet or gentian violet solution (0.5% solution)

1. Dissolve 5 gm of methyl violet **or** crystal violet **or** gentian violet powder in 1000 ml of distilled water.
2. Filter, store at room temperature in stoppered glass bottle with label (0.5% methyl violet or 0.5% crystal violet or 0.5% gentian violet, depending on the stain used), date of preparation and expiry date of one year.

Mordant: Gram's Iodine

1. Grind 1.0 g of iodine crystal and 2.0 g of potassium iodide in a mortar.
2. Add water slowly with continuous grinding until iodine is dissolved.
3. Make up the volume to 300 ml. Filter. **Store** at room temperature in **amber coloured** bottles **with label, date of preparation and expiry date of 6 months.**

Decolouriser: Acetone–Alcohol

1. Mix 400 ml of reagent grade acetone with 400 ml of 95% ethanol.
2. Store at room temperature in stoppered brown bottle with label (acetone – alcohol decolouriser), date of preparation and expiry date of six months.

Counterstain: 0.5% Safranin Solution or 0.2% Basic Fuchsin Solution

0.5% Safranin Solution

1. Dissolve 5 gm of safranin powder in 1000 ml of distilled water.
2. Filter, store at room temperature in stoppered brown glass bottle with label (0.5% safranin solution), date of preparation and expiry date of one year.

0.2% Basic Fuchsin Solution

1. Dissolve 2 g of basic fuchsin powder in 1000 ml of distilled water.
2. Filter, store at room temperature in stoppered brown glass bottle with label (0.2% basic fuchsin solution), date of preparation and expiry date of one year.

12.7 PROCEDURE

12.7.1 Preparation of Smear

Make a thin smear on a clean slide from agar or broth culture of known organisms.

In case of making smear from different clinical specimens, prepare a thicker smear with specific instructions as under:

- For **pus or similar exudates**, spread the sample on the slide with sterile needle or applicator stick over an area of 2 cm × 1 cm approximately.
- For **wet swabs**, roll the swabs on the slide to make a smear.

- For **swabs containing dried materials**, roll the swab on a drop of saline placed on the slide.
- For **sputum,** make the smear with of blood tinged particles, if present.
- For **faeces**, make the smear with the mucus or blood, if present in the stool specimen.
- For **centrifuged specimen**, use a sterile, capillary pipette with a rubber bulb to collect the drop and use the tip of the pipette to spread the drop to an even film of proper density.

12.7.2 Staining

1. Heat fix the smear.
2. Cover the heat fixed smear with the primary stain (methyl violet or crystal violet or gentian violet).
3. Allow the stain to remain for 30 seconds.
4. Wash with water.
5. Flood the smear with Gram's iodine for 30 seconds.
6. Rinse gently with running tap water.
7. Add acetone–alcohol decolouriser over the smear dropwise holding the slide in a slanting position.
8. Stop decolourisation as soon as the dripping solution from the slide becomes clear.
9. Remove the excess decolouriser with a gentle flow of water.
10. Apply the counter stain, i.e. safranin or basic fuchsin for 30 seconds.
11. Hold the slide under a gentle flow of tap water.
12. Drain the slide and air dry.
13. Add a drop of immersion oil on the smear and observe the smear under the microscope with the oil immersion objective (Fig. 12.2).

12.8 OBSERVATION

- All Gram-positive organisms including yeast cells shall appear purple (Fig. 12.3).
- Gram-negative organisms shall appear red (Fig. 12.3).
- Pus cells and epithelial cells will appear red.
- Granules, if present, take up the stain more strongly than the remaining part of the bacteria (Fig. 12.4).
- In spore bearing bacteria, endospores are seen as colourless regions within the stained cells (Fig. 12.5).
- Nuclei of the epithelial cells and WBCs shall appear dark red (Fig. 12.6).

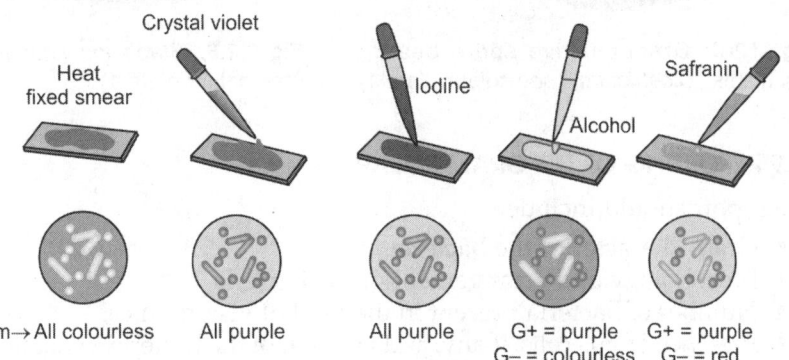

Fig. 12.2: Colour taken by the Gram-positive and Gram-negative organisms during and after Gram staining

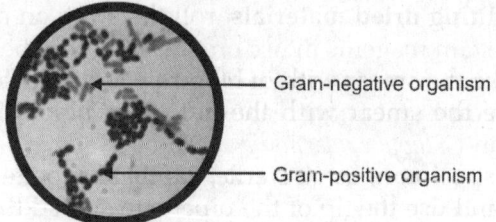

Fig. 12.3: Gram-positive and Gram-negative organisms (*see* colour plate 1)

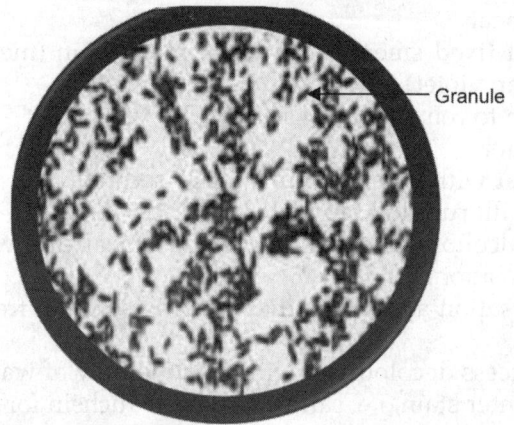

Fig. 12.4: Gram-positive organism (diphtheria bacillus) with granules (*see* colour plate 1)

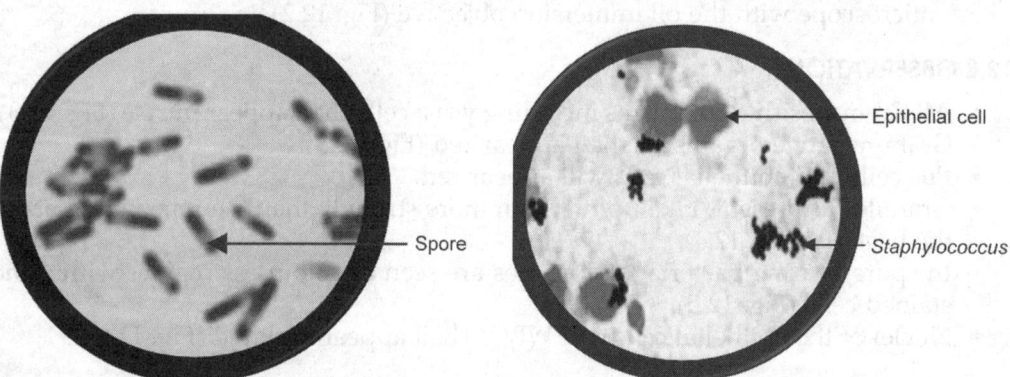

Fig. 12.5: Gram-positive spore bearing organisms (*Clostridium*) (*see* colour plate 1)

Fig. 12.6: *Staphylococcus* in a sputum sample (*see* colour plate 1)

12.9 REPORTING OF THE GRAM SMEAR

The report should include:

- Gram character of the bacteria.
- Morphology and arrangement of the bacteria.
- Number of bacteria present in the field of vision (in case of specimens like CSF).
- Presence of pus cells, if any, and position of the bacteria in relation to the pus cells.
- Presence and position of endospore or volutin granules, if any, inside Gram-positive rods.

12.10 QUALITY CONTROL

- Check the Gram stain reagents in use on the laboratory bench at least once daily.
- Stain the control smears of *Escherichia coli* and *Staphylococcus epidermidis* following the staining procedures mentioned above. *Escherichia coli* should be seen as Gram-negative bacilli and *Staph. epidermidis* should be seen as Gram-positive cocci.

12.11 LABORATORY RECORD

Perform Gram staining with different specimens or with pure culture of organisms. Record your observations.

Date	Name of the organism/specimen	Observation				Teacher's signature
		Gram character	Shape	Arrangement	Special character-istics, if any	

13

Ziehl-Neelsen Staining

13.1 AIM

To make the students understand the meaning of Ziehl-Neelsen staining or acid fast staining, the importance of Ziehl-Neelsen staining for identification of the causative agents of tuberculosis and leprosy and the correct method to carry out the staining method.

13.2 LEARNING OUTCOME

After this session, the students understand the importance and meaning of acid fast staining and learn to perform Ziehl-Neelsen staining following universal precautions.

13.3 PURPOSE

Ziehl-Neelsen staining or acid fast staining is a method for identification of the bacilli responsible for tuberculosis and leprosy. Acid fast staining is also used for identification of *Nocardia* and spores.

13.4 PRINCIPLE

Bacteria causing tuberculosis (*Mycobacterium tuberculosis*) and leprosy (*Mycobacterium leprae*), have cell walls where the peptidoglycan is cross linked with a complex waxy lipid (waxy material) called mycolic acid (Fig. 13.1). This waxy layer makes the organisms resistant to ordinary staining methods. These organisms are stained only with drastic methods and once stained, are able to retain the dye despite washing with acid or acid alcohol mixture. Therefore, this staining method is also known as acid fast staining and the organisms are called acid fast organisms. Acid fastness depends are on the structural integrity of the cells.

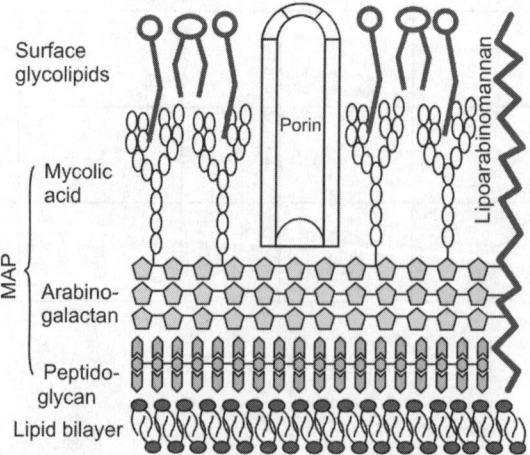

Fig. 13.1: Cell wall structure of acid fast bacilli

13.5 MATERIALS REQUIRED

13.5.1 Specimen

- For *Mycobacterium tuberculosis:* Sputum, gastric lavage, urine, tissues, other body fluids.
- For *Mycobacterium leprae,* nasal scraping or sample from skin lesion.

13.5.2 Reagents

1. **Primary stain:** (0.3% carbol fuchsin solution).
2. **Decolourising agent:** Conc. of hydrochloric acid—ethyl alcohol or sulphuric acid.
3. **Counterstain:** 0.3% methylene blue solution or 0.5% malachite green solution.

13.6 PREPARATION OF REAGENTS

Primary stain: Carbol fuchsin solution.

Ingredients: Basic fuchsin, 95% ethanol, phenol crystals.

Preparation of Carbol Fuchsin

1. Dissolve 0.3 gm of basic fuchsin in 10 ml of 95% ethyl alcohol.
2. Melt 5 gm of phenol crystal with gentle heat, dissolve it in 100 ml of water.
3. Mix 10 ml of fuchsin solution with 90 ml of the phenol solution.
4. Filter, store at room temperature in stoppered brown glass bottle with label (i.e. carbol fuchsin solution), date of preparation and expiry date.

Composition of Decolourising Agent (Acid or Acid Alcohol)

- For *M. tuberculosis*: 20% sulphuric acid or 3% acid alcohol.
- For *M. leprae:* 5% sulphuric acid or 0.5% acid alcohol.
- For Nocardia: 1% sulphuric acid.
- For spores: 0.25% – 0.5% sulphuric acid.

Preparation of Decolourising Agents

- **20% sulphuric acid:** very slowly add 20 ml concentrated sulphuric acid (98%) – 80 ml of distilled water and mix gently. **Never add water to acid.**
- **3% acid alcohol:** Carefully add 3 ml of concentrated hydrochloric acid to 97 ml of 95% ethyl alcohol and mix gently.
- **5% sulphuric acid:** slowly add 5 ml concentrated sulphuric acid to 95 ml of distilled water and mix gently.
- **1% sulphuric acid:** slowly add 1 ml concentrated sulphuric acid to 99 ml of distilled water and mix gently.
- **0.5% sulphuric acid:** slowly add 0.5 ml concentrated sulphuric acid to 99.5 ml of distilled water and mix gently.
- **0.5% acid alcohol:** add 0.5 ml of concentrated hydrochloric acid to 99.5 ml of 95% ethyl alcohol and mix gently.

Store the reagents in stoppered glass bottle with label appropriately with name, date of preparation and expiry date.

Counter stain: 0.3% methylene blue solution or 0.5% malachite green solution

0.3% methylene blue solution

Dissolve 0.3 g methylene blue chloride in 100 ml distilled water. Filter and store in stoppered bottle with proper labeling.

0.5% malachite green solution

Dissolve 0.5 g malachite green in 100 ml distilled water. Filter and store in stoppered bottle with proper labeling.

13.7 PROCEDURE FOR ACID FAST STAINING

- Prepare a thick smear by spreading the specimen over an area of 1 × 2 cm on a scratch free slide. Select the cheesy or necrotic blood tinged part of the material from the specimen, wherever available.
- Heat fix by using a slide warmer or a Bunsen flame. Do not overheat.
- Place a rectangular (2 × 3 cm) filter paper on the slide covering the smear. Add enough carbol fuchsin to flood the filter paper completely or add freshly filtered carbol fuchsin.
- Place the slide on a beaker containing boiling water for 8 minutes or gently heat the bottom of the slide by the Bunsen flame until steam begins to rise. Let it stand for 5 minutes without additional heating. Do not boil or allow the stain to dry. Add more staining reagent on the filter paper if necessary, but do not reheat.
- Remove the filter strips with forceps. Discard in the discarding jar.
- Wash the slide with water.
- Based on the organism to be identified (i.e. *M. tuberculosis* or *M. leprae, or Nocardia or spores*), select the concentration of the decolourising agent and de-stain the smear for 15–20 seconds.
- Wash the smear with water and drain.
- Flood smear with the counter stain (i.e. methylene blue or malachite green). Allow to act for 30 seconds.
- Rinse the smear with water, drain and air dry (Fig. 13.2).
- Examine the smear under oil immersion objective. While examining the smear for tubercle bacilli, ensure that the entire smear is searched for the acid fast bacilli in an orderly manner by making a series of three horizontal or nine vertical sweeps (Fig. 13.3). If the smear is heavily positive, then fewer fields may be examined.

13.8 OBSERVATION

Tubercle bacilli, leprosy bacilli, spore and other acid fast bacilli are red. Non-acid fast cells appear as blue or green depending on the counter stain used (Fig. 13.4 for tubercle bacilli and Fig. 13.5 for leprosy bacilli).

13.9 REPORTING

For *Mycobacterium tuberculosis*

- Report only the number of acid fast bacilli seen under the microscope under the oil immersion objective. Do not try to identify the organism by microscopy alone.
- Report large number of clumps, if any.
- For sputum, the CDC recommends the following method of reporting.

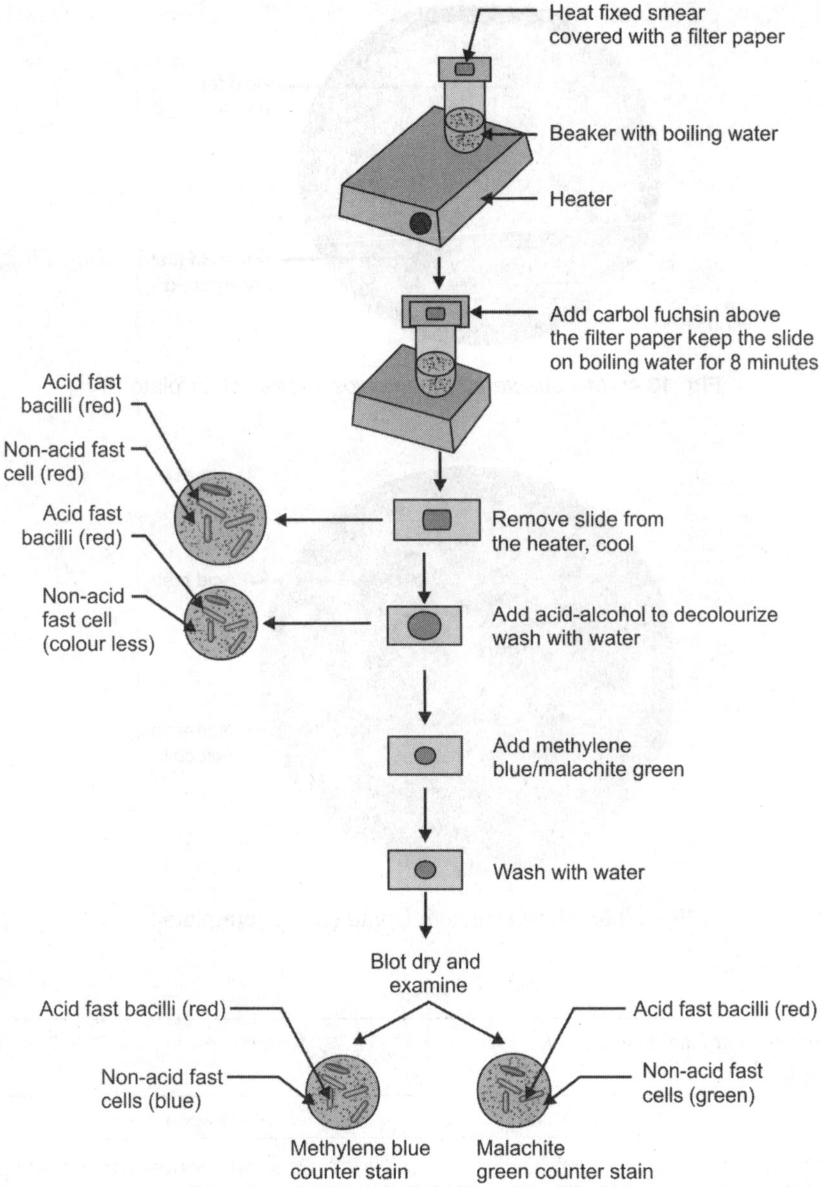

Heat fixed smear
covered with a filter paper

Beaker with boiling water

Heater

Add carbol fuchsin above
the filter paper keep the slide
on boiling water for 8 minutes

Acid fast
bacilli (red)

Non-acid fast
cell (red)

Acid fast
bacilli (red)

Remove slide from
the heater, cool

Non-acid
fast cell
(colour less)

Add acid-alcohol to decolourize
wash with water

Add methylene
blue/malachite green

Wash with water

Blot dry and
examine

Acid fast bacilli (red)

Non-acid fast
cells (blue)

Methylene blue
counter stain

Acid fast bacilli (red)

Non-acid fast
cells (green)

Malachite
green counter stain

Fig. 13.2: Acid fast staining procedure

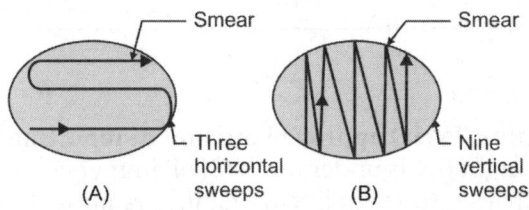

Smear

Smear

Three
horizontal
sweeps

Nine
vertical
sweeps

(A)

(B)

Figs 13.3 (A and B): Recommended method for examining acid fast smear for tubercle bacilli (A) Three horizontal sweeps (B) Nine vertical sweeps

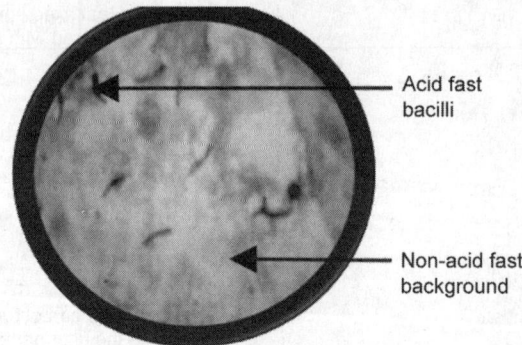

Fig. 13.4: *Mycobacterium tuberculosis* (*see* colour plate 2)

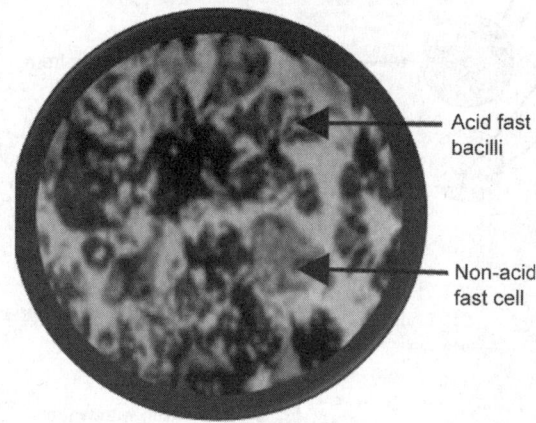

Fig. 13.5: *Mycobacterium leprae* (*see* colour plate 2)

Number of acid fast bacilli seen in oil immersion field	Report
None	No AFB seen
1–2/300 fields	±, send request for repeat specimen
1–9/100 fields	1 +
1–9/10 fields	2 +
1–9/field	3 +
> 9/field	4 +

For Mycobacterium Leprae

For skin or nasal scraping, WHO approved method of reporting the bacteriological index is to count six to eight fields under the 100X oil immersion lens in a smear made by nicking the skin with a sharp scalpel, scraping it, spreading the fluid and the tissue fairly thickly on a slide and staining by the Ziehl-Neelsen method and decolourizing with 1% acid alcohol. The results are expressed on a logarithmic scale.

Number of acid fast bacilli seen	Report/bacteriological index
Nil in the entire smear	No AFB seen
At least 1 AFB in every 100 fields	1 +
At least 1 AFB in every 10 fields	2 +
At least 1 AFB in every field	3 +
At least 10 AFB in every field	4 +
At least 100 AFB in every field	5 +
At least 1000 AFB in every field	6 +

13.10 QUALITY CONTROL

- Use new slides free from scratches.
- Use acid fast bacilli free water.
- Use known acid fast positive sputum or tissue for checking the reagents.
- Use negative controls to ensure that acid fast contaminants are not present in the staining solutions or in water.
- Get positive smears confirmed by a second reader also.

13.11 LABORATORY RECORDS

Perform acid fast staining with various specimens. Record your observation as under

Date	Specimen	Report	Teacher's signature

14

Albert Staining

14.1 AIM

To demonstrate the presumptive diagnosis of diphtheria through Albert staining method.

14.2 LEARNING OBJECTIVE

Students learn to perform Albert's staining and to identify volutin granules or metachromatic granules.

14.3 PURPOSE

Albert staining is used for preliminary identification of diphtheria bacilli.

14.4 PRINCIPLE

Diphtheria bacillus contains energy rich polymetaphosphate granules (also called volutin granules or metachromatic granules), which, when stained, shows a colour that is different from the colour of the stain used. Albert staining demonstrates the presence of volutin granules that are best observed in a young culture of diphtheria bacilli on a blood or serum containing medium.

14.5 MATERIALS REQUIRED

- Culture of diphtheria bacilli/specimen from throat.
- Toluidine blue, malachite green, glacial acetic acid, 95% ethanol, and distilled water to make Albert's stain 1.
- Iodine, potassium iodide and distilled water to make Albert stain II (Albert's iodine.)
- Slides.

14.6 PREPARATION OF REAGENTS

Ingredients for Albert's stain I

- Toluidine blue 1.5 g
- Malachite green 2 g
- Glacial acetic acid 10 ml
- 95% ethanol 20 ml
- Distilled water 1000 ml

Preparation of Albert stain 1: Dissolve the dyes in alcohol, add to acid-water mixture allow to stand for 1 day, filter, store in stoppered bottles with proper label regarding the name of the reagent, date of preparation and expiry date.

Ingredients of Albert stain II (Albert's iodine)
- Iodine 2 gm
- Potassium iodide 3 gm
- Distilled water 300 ml

Preparation

Dissolve the potassium iodide in a small volume of water, add iodine with gentle shaking. Make up the volume to 300 ml.

14.7 PROCEDURE
- Prepare heat fixed smear on a clean, grease free slide.
- Cover the smear with Albert's stain I for 3 minutes.
- Wash with water.
- Cover with Albert's iodine for 1 minute.
- Wash with water, air dry and examine under oil immersion objective.

14.8 RESULT

Volutin granules bluish black, protoplasm of the organism green and other organisms light green (Fig. 14.1).

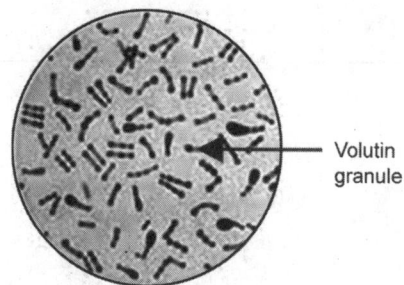

Volutin granule

Fig. 14.1: *Corynebacterium diphtheriae* as seen after Albert staining (*see* colour plate 2)

14.9 REPORT

Indicate whether the volutin granules are present or absent.

14.10 QUALITY CONTROL
- Use known positive and negative controls to check the strains.
- Ensure that young culture of *Corynebacterium diphtheriae* is used as a positive control.
- Get the positive slides checked by a second person.

14.11 LABORATORY RECORD

Perform Albert staining. Record your observation:

Date	Name of the organism/specimen	Observation	Teacher's signature

15

Capsule Staining

15.1 AIM

To demonstrate bacterial capsules by negative staining, i.e., staining the background instead of the organism.

15.2 LEARNING OUTCOME

After completing the exercise, the students shall be able to perform negative staining and to observe the bacterial capsules.

15.3 PRINCIPLE

Bacterial capsule is a rigid, viscous layer surrounding the cell walls of some of the pathogenic bacteria (Fig. 15.1). Capsule is visible with negative staining, in which the background is stained with an acidic dye or with a combination of direct staining and negative staining.

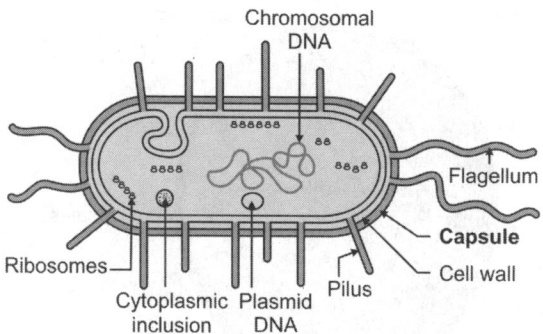

Fig. 15.1: Position of capsule in relation to bacterial structure

15.4 METHODS

Two methods are used for demonstrating capsules:

1. Negative staining method in which an acidic dye or a dye of large particle size is chosen. Bacterial cell and capsule does not take the stain. Only background becomes coloured.
2. Combination of negative staining and direct staining. The capsule remains colourless in between the stained bacterial cell and coloured background.

15.4.1 Materials Required

- Slide
- Coverslip

- Bacterial culture.
- Inoculating loop.
- India ink (for negative staining).
- Safranin, 6% dextrose solution, alcohol (for combination of negative staining and direct staining).

15.5 PROCEDURE

15.5.1 Negative Staining

1. Take a clean grease free slide.
2. Place a drop of India ink at the centre of the slide.
3. Aseptically pick up a small portion of bacterial culture and mix it with the India ink.
4. Cover with a cover slip ensuring that no air bubble is trapped between the slide and the coverslip.
5. Place the slide–cover slip combination between two pieces of blotting paper and press to have a light coloured film between the slide and the cover slip.
6. Examine under oil immersion objective.

Observation: The capsulated bacteria appears to be surrounded by a clear zone against a dark gray background (Fig. 15.2).

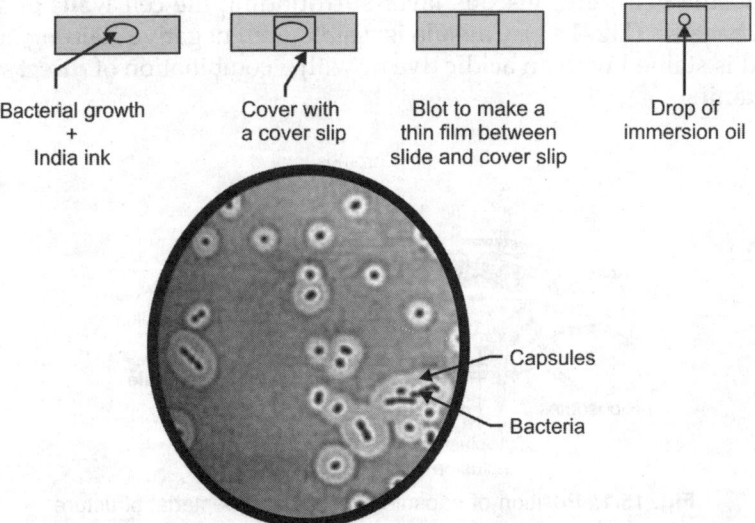

Bacterial growth + India ink | Cover with a cover slip | Blot to make a thin film between slide and cover slip | Drop of immersion oil

Capsules

Bacteria

Fig. 15.2: Visualization of capsules by negative staining

15.5.2 Combination of Negative Staining and Direct Staining (Fig. 15.3)

1. Place several loopfuls of bacterial culture on one side of a grease free slide.
2. Add equal volume of India ink near the culture drop without touching the culture. Add one drop of 6% dextrose solution to make the capsule larger.
3. Mix the liquids and spread the mixture along the side following blood smear technique.
4. Air dry the smear.
5. Fix by dipping the slide in alcohol contained in a beaker.
6. Drain the slide dry.

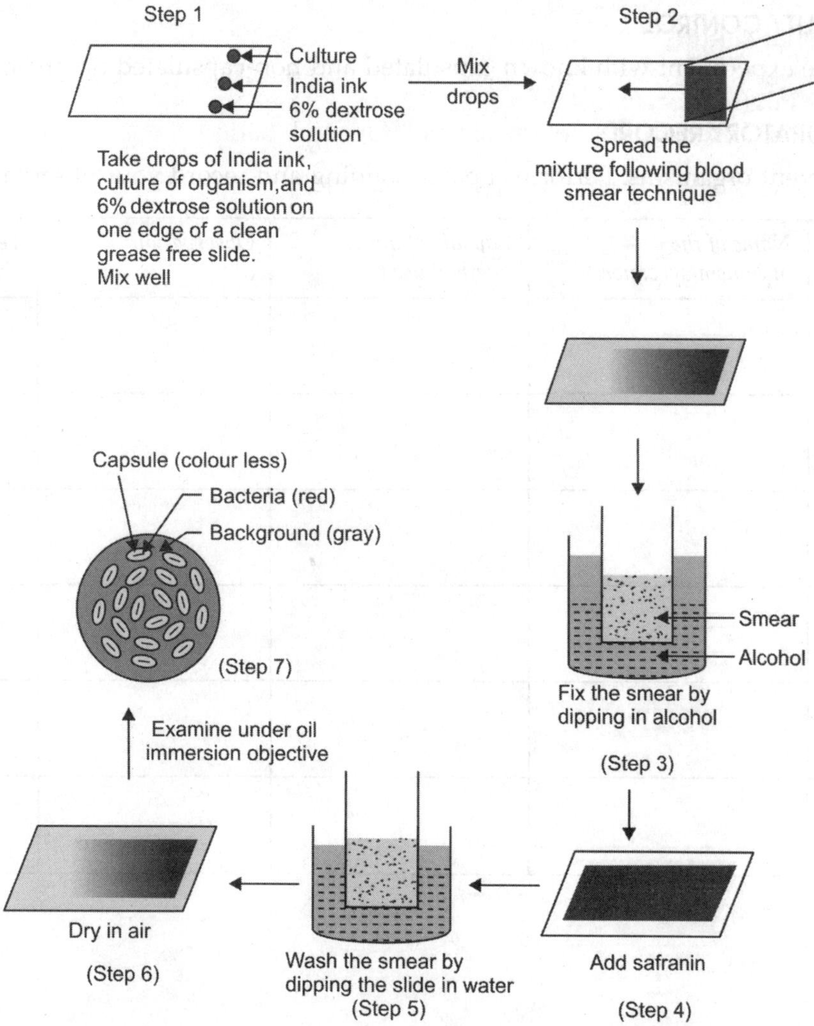

Step 1

Culture
India ink
6% dextrose solution

Mix drops

Take drops of India ink, culture of organism, and 6% dextrose solution on one edge of a clean grease free slide. Mix well

Step 2

Spread the mixture following blood smear technique

Smear

Alcohol

Fix the smear by dipping in alcohol

(Step 3)

Add safranin

(Step 4)

Wash the smear by dipping the slide in water

(Step 5)

Dry in air

(Step 6)

Examine under oil immersion objective

Capsule (colour less)

Bacteria (red)

Background (gray)

(Step 7)

Fig. 15.3: Method of viewing capsules using a combination of negative staining and direct staining

6. Cover the smear with 0.5% safranin solution for 10 seconds.
7. Wash the excess stain by dipping the slide in a beaker of distilled water.
8. Drain dry.

Observation (Fig. 15.4)
- Bacteria: red.
- Capsule: colourless.
- Background dark gray.

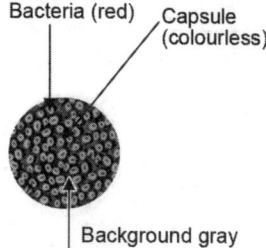

Bacteria (red)   Capsule (colourless)

Background gray

Fig. 15.4: Visualization of capsule after staining the cell with safranin and background with India ink (*see* colour plate 2)

15.6 QUALITY CONTROL

Repeat the experiment with known capsulated and non-capsulated organisms.

15.7 LABORATORY RECORD

Take different organisms. Perform capsule staining and record your observation:

Date	Name of the organism/specimen	Capsule staining method used	Observation	Teacher's signature

Preparation of Various Culture Media

16.1 AIM

To explain the importance of growing organisms in artificial nutrient medium (pleural media) towards their further isolation and identification and to demonstrate the preparation of various culture media.

16.2 LEARNING OUTCOME

The students can make different solid and liquid nutrient preparations (called culture media) in sterile conditions using appropriate methods of sterilization and learn the use(s) of each medium prepared.

16.3 PURPOSE

Culture media are prepared for cultivation of the organisms in the laboratory for their subsequent isolation in pure culture, identification by their growth characteristics and biochemical reaction and to determine their susceptibility against different antibiotics.

Most of the microbiology laboratories now use readymade culture media.

16.4 PRINCIPLE

Nutrients for preparing culture media for growing an organism are chosen on the basis of the growth requirement and energy requirement of the particular organism intended to grow.

- **Nutrients for growth requirement**
  - **Organic sources:** Nitrogen containing compounds, e.g. proteins and their breakdown products and other accessory growth factors.
  - **Inorganic sources:** Inorganic salts, essential elements and trace elements.
- **Nutrients for energy requirement**
  - **Organic sources:** Usually carbohydrates of varying degrees of complexity. Protein, in absence of available carbohydrates, are also used by certain organisms.
  - **Inorganic sources:** Various energy rich inorganic molecules, e.g. phosphates.
- Water
- Agar-agar to make the medium solid or semisolid.

16.5 MATERIALS REQUIRED

- Required nitrogen and energy sources.
- Analytical balance with weight box.
- pH meter/pH comparator/pH paper.
- Water

- N/10 and 10N sodium hydroxide (NaOH) solution for adjusting the pH.
- Agar-agar powder.
- Autoclave for sterilization.

16.6 GENERAL METHOD OF PREPARATION OF A CULTURE MEDIUM

16.6.1 Weigh the Ingredients

Take the ingredients for the particular culture medium you intend to prepare and according to the standard composition of the medium, weigh the ingredients in a container.

16.6.2 Dissolve the Ingredients in Water

- For preparing a liquid medium (broth), dissolve the easily soluble ingredients in a small volume of water with gentle heating, if required. Make up the volume with more water.
- For preparing an agar medium, dissolve agar-agar in the liquid medium using a water bath at a temperature more than 80°C. Continuously stir the suspension to avoid concentrated heating and subsequent charring of agar.

16.6.3 Adjust the pH to 7.4

Calculation for pH adjustment: If 5 ml of the medium requires X ml of N/10 NaOH for raising the pH to 7.4, 1000 ml of the medium shall require 1000/5=200X ml of N/10 NaOH for raising the pH to 7.4, i.e. 20X ml of N NaOH or 2X ml of 10N NaOH. Minimum volume of NaOH has to be added to the preparation to minimize changes in the concentration of the nutrients in the prepared medium.

16.6.4 Filtration

Filter the medium through filter paper for liquid medium. In case of agar medium, filter the molten hot agar through layers of gauge piece or cheese cloth.

16.6.5. Distribution and Sterilization

16.6.5.1 Medium Containing Heat Stable Materials

- Distribute the medium containing heat stable materials in clean, unsterile glass tubes or bottles without taking sterile precautions, filling not more than 75% from the bottom.
- Sterilize the media in the autoclave at specified temperature or pressure.

16.6.5.2 Medium Containing Heat Labile Materials

- Sterilize the heat labile ingredients by suitable methods, e.g. filtration.
- Add this sterile heat labile material to the main sterile medium with aseptic precautions after proper cooling.
- Distribute aseptically into sterile containers.

16.6.6 Quality Control

- Check the sterility of the prepared medium by incubating samples from the autoclaved and distributed samples.
- Check the ingredients by inoculating known organisms in or on the culture medium and see their growth.
- Check the autoclave functioning by using packets of *Bacillus stearothermophilus* or by indicator tapes.

16.7 PREPARATION OF COMMON CULTURE MEDIA USED IN A ROUTINE MICROBIOLOGY LABORATORY

16.7.1 Liquid Medium or Broth

16.7.1.1 Peptone Water Medium

Uses:
- For rapid growth of non-fastidious organisms.
- As a base for making other media.
- For performing certain biochemical tests.
- For preparing the inoculum for antibiotic sensitivity test.

Ingredient	Method of preparation
• Peptone 10 g (**always close the mouth of the bottle tightly after each use**) • Sodium chloride 5 g • Distilled water 1 litre	1. Weigh the ingredients. 2. Dissolve the ingredients in a small volume of water. 3. Make up the volume of the medium to 1 litre. 4. Adjust the pH to 7.3 and 7.4. 5. Filter the medium. 6. Distribute in tubes. 7. Sterilize by autoclaving at 15 lbs pressure for 18 minutes. 8. Cool and store at 4°C.

16.7.1.2 Glucose Phosphate Peptone Water Medium

Use: For observing the metabolic end products of glucose utilization for preliminary identification of organisms.

Ingredient	Method of preparation
• Peptone 5 g • Dipotassium hydrogen phosphate 5 g • Glucose 5 g • Distilled water 1 litre	Follow similar steps as that for preparation of peptone water up to the sterilization step. Sterilize by autoclaving at 8 lbs pressure for 30 minutes to prevent charring of glucose. Cool and store at 4°C.

16.7.1.3 Nutrient Broth Medium (Meat Extract Broth)

Uses:
- For growth of non-fastidious organisms
- As a basal medium used for making enriched broths like glucose broth, serum broth, etc.

Ingredient	Method of preparation
• Peptone 10 g • Meat extract 10 g • Sodium chloride 5 g • Distilled water 1 litre	1. Weigh the ingredients. 2. Dissolve the peptone and sodium chloride in a small volume of water. 3. Add meat extract and dissolve by gentle heating. 4. Make up the volume of the medium to 1 litre. 5. Adjust the pH to 7.2 to 7.4. 6. Filter the medium. 7. Distribute in bottles and into tubes (not more than 75% from the bottom of the container. 8. Sterilize by autoclaving at 15 lbs pressure for 15–18 minutes. 9. Cool and store at 4°C.

16.7.1.4 Glucose Broth

Use: As an enriched medium for growing *Streptococcus* and other Gram-positive bacteria.

Ingredient	Method of preparation
• Nutrient broth 100 ml • Glucose 1 g	1. Dissolve glucose in nutrient broth. 2. Distribute in tubes. 3. Sterilize at 10 lbs pressure for 45 minutes. 4. Cool and store at 4°C.

16.7.2 Solid Medium

16.7.2.1. Nutrient Agar Medium

Uses

- For growth of non-fastidious organisms and for examination of the colony characteristics.
- As a base for making enriched media, e.g. blood agar medium, serum agar medium, etc.
- For better visualization of colours produced by pigment producing organisms.

Ingredient	Method of preparation
• Peptone 10 g • Meat extract 10 g • Sodium chloride 5 g • Distilled water 1 litre • Agar agar 15–20 g	1. Follow the steps as described for nutrient broth. 2. Add agar-agar. Dissolve the agar by free steaming or by continuous stirring by placing the container in a hot water bath. 3. Filter through layers of gauge piece while the preparation is very hot. 4. Distribute in bottles. 5. Sterilize by autoclaving at 15 lbs pressure for 15 minutes. 6. For pouring plates, cool the sterile molten media at an approximate temperature of 52°C. 7. Distribute the sterile medium in sterile petridishes with sterile precautions. 8. Store at 4°C.

16.7.2.2. Blood Agar Medium

Uses

- An enriched medium. It facilitates growth of almost all organisms.
- Used for seeing the hemolytic properties of the organisms.
- Also used for seeing swarming growth of motile organisms.

Ingredient	Method of preparation and distribution
• Sterile nutrient agar 100 ml • Blood 5–50% (Usually 10%) collected with aseptic precautions from sheep.	**Single layer blood agar medium** 1. Melt sterile nutrient agar. 2. Cool to about 50–52°C. 3. Add sterile blood with sterile precaution. 4. Mix slowly.

(Contd.)

(Contd.)

Ingredient	Method of preparation and distribution
	5. Pour immediately into sterile petridishes.
	6. Allow to solidify.
	7. Store at 4°C.
	Double layered blood agar medium
	(helps in better visualization of hemolysis)
	1. Take petri dishes of 100 mm × 15mm size.
	2. Pour approximately 7 ml of sterile molten nutrient agar.
	3. Allow the nutrient agar to solidify.
	4. Pour approx 7 ml of 10% blood agar medium to make a thin layer on the nutrient agar.
	5. Allow the blood agar to solidify.
	6. Store at 4°C.

Quality Control

- Check the sterility of the blood agar medium by keeping one plate in the incubator for overnight. There should not be any growth after incubation.
- Check the ingredients by inoculating one plate with *Streptococcus pyogenes*. There should be good growth with clear hemolysis around the colonies.

16.7.2.3 Chocolate Agar (CHOC) or Chocolate Blood Agar (CBA)

Uses

- As a non-selective, enriched medium for growth of fastidious organisms as it contains nicotinamide adenine dinucleotide (NAD) and hemin released from lysis of the red blood cells by slow heating of blood at 80°C.
- Can be made selective for *Haemophilus* by addition of bacitracin and for *Neisseria* by adding a group of different antibiotics.

Preparation

1. Melt required volume of sterile nutrient agar base in a steamer or water bath.
2. Slowly heat 10% of fresh sheep blood at 80°C till it is hemolysed.
3. Add to the molten agar medium.
4. Mix well, immediately pour into sterile petridishes.
5. Store at 4–8°C.

16.7.2.4 MacConkey's Medium

Uses

- As a selective medium for growth of intestinal organisms.
- To isolate intestinal organisms.
- As an indicator medium to see the lactose fermenting ability of the intestinal organisms.

Ingredient	Method of preparation
• Peptone 20 g • Commercial sodium taurocholate 5 g • Distilled water 1 litre • Agar-agar 20 g • Neutral red (2% in 50% ethyl alcohol) Approx 3.5 ml • Lactose 10 g	1. Weigh the ingredients. 2. Dissolve peptone and sodium taurocholate in water by gentle heating. 3. Make up the volume of the medium to 1 litre. 4. Filter. 5. Adjust the pH to 7.5. 6. Add agar-agar. Dissolve the agar by free steaming or by continuous stirring by placing the container in a water bath. 7. Add lactose and neutral red. 8. Check the colour of the medium by allowing a small quantity of the medium to solidify. If required, add a little more neutral red. 9. Distribute in bottles. 10. Sterilize by autoclaving at 8 lbs pressure for 30 minutes. 11. Cool a part of the sterile molten media to an approximate temperature of 52°C. 12. Distribute this cooled sterile medium in sterile petridishes with sterile precautions. Remaining sterile medium can be stored in the bottles. 13. Store at 4°C.

Quality Control

- Check the sterility of the MacConkey agar medium by keeping one plate in the incubator for overnight. There should not be any growth after incubation.
- Check the ingredients by inoculating one plate with known lactose fermenting and known non-lactose fermenting organisms. There should be good growth with magenta colonies of lactose fermenting organisms and pale colonies of non-lactose fermenting organisms.

16.7.2.5 Xylose Lysine Deoxycholate Agar (XLD Agar) Medium

Use: Isolation and preliminary identification of *Salmonella* and *Shigella* species from clinical samples and from food.

Ingredient	Method of preparation
• Yeast extract 3 g • L-lysine 5 g • Xylose 3.75 g • Lactose 7.5 g • Sucrose 7.5 g • Sodium deoxycholate 1 g • Sodium chloride 5 g • Sodium thiosulfate 6.8 g • Ferric ammonium citrate 0.8 g • Phenol red 0.08 g • Agar 12.5 g • Distilled water 1 litre	1. Weigh the ingredients. 2. Dissolve the ingredients by heating with constant agitation until the medium starts boiling. Do not overheat. 3. Transfer immediately to a water bath and cool to 50°C. 4. Pour plates as soon as the medium has cooled. 5. Store the prepared medium up to 30 days protected from light at 2–8°C 6. Final pH, 7.4 ± 0.2. Warning: The medium is heat sensitive. No further sterilization is necessary or desirable.

16.7.2.6 Triple Sugar Iron Medium

Use: For preliminary identification of intestinal organisms.

Ingredient	Method of preparation
• Beef extract 3.0 g • Yeast extract 3.0 g • Peptone 15 g • Proteose peptone 5 g • Lactose 10.0 g • Sucrose 10 g • Glucose 1 g • Ferrous sulphate 0.2 g • Sodium chloride 5 g • Sodium thiosulphate 0.3 g • Phenol red 0.024 g • Agar 12 g • Distilled water 1 litre	1. Weigh the ingredients. 2. Dissolve the ingredients except agar-agar in water by gentle heating. 3. Make up the volume of the medium to 1 litre. 4. Adjust the pH to 7.2 to 7.4. 5. Add agar-agar. Dissolve the agar by free steaming or by continuous stirring by placing the container in a water bath . 6. Filter through layers of gauge piece while the preparation is very hot. 7. Distribute in bottles/tubes. 8. Sterilize by autoclaving at 8 lbs pressure for 30 minutes. 9. Allow the media solidify in the tubes as agar slants. 10. Store at 4°C.

16.7.2.7 Simmon's Citrate Medium

Uses: For preliminary identification of organisms by observing the organism's ability to use citrate as a sole carbon and energy source for growth.

Ingredient	Method of preparation
• Sodium chloride 5 g • Magnesium sulphate 0.2 g • Ammonium dihydrogen phosphate 1.0 g • Potassium dihydrogen phosphate 1.0 g • Sodium citrate 5 g • Distilled water 1 litre • Agar-agar 20 g • Bromothymol blue (1 g in 25 ml of 0.1N NaOH) −40 ml	1. Weigh the ingredients. 2. Dissolve the ingredients in water by gentle heating. 3. Make up the volume of the medium to 1 litre. 4. Adjust the pH to 6.8. 5. Add agar-agar. Dissolve the agar by free steaming or by continuous stirring by placing the container in a water bath. 6. Filter through layers of gauge piece. 7. Distribute in tubes. 8. Sterilize by autoclaving at 15 lbs pressure for 15–18 minutes. 9. Allow to solidify as agar slants in test tubes. 10. Store at 4°C.

Quality Control

- Check the sterility of the prepared medium by keeping one tube in the incubator for overnight. There should not be any growth after incubation.
- Check the ingredients by inoculating one tube with known citrate utilizing organism. There should be good surface growth with blue colour around the growth.

16.7.2.8 Christensen's Urease Medium

Use: An indicator medium for preliminary identification of urease producing bacteria.

Ingredient	Method of preparation
• Peptone 0.1 g • Sodium chloride 0.5 g • Dipotassium hydrogen phosphate 0.2 g • Distilled water 100 ml • Agar-agar 2 g • Phenol red (1 in 500 aq solution) 0.6 ml • Sterile 10% glucose solution 1 ml • Sterile 20% urea solution 10 ml	1. Weigh the ingredients. 2. Dissolve the ingredients (except glucose and urea) in distilled water. 3. Adjust the pH to 6.8. 4. Add agar-agar. Dissolve the agar by free steaming or by continuous stirring by placing the container in a water bath. 5. Filter through layers of gauge piece. 6. Sterilize the basal medium by autoclaving at 15 lbs pressure for 15–18 minutes. 7. Sterilize the glucose solution and the urea solution by filtration. 8. Cool the molten agar medium to 50°C. 9. Add sterile glucose and sterile urea solution. 10. Mix well by gentle mixing. 11. Pour aseptically in sterile tubes. 12. Store at 4°C.

Quality Control

- Check the sterility of the prepared medium by keeping one tube in the incubator for overnight. There should not be any growth after incubation.
- Check the ingredients by inoculating one tube with known urease producing organism. There should be good growth with red colour around the growth.

16.7.2.9 Hugh and Leifson Medium

Uses:
- To view utilization of various carbohydrates by different organisms.
- To differentiate between oxidative utilization and fermentative utilization of various carbohydrates.

Ingredient	Method of preparation
• Peptone 0.2 g • Sodium chloride 0.5 g • Dipotassium hydrogen phosphate 0.03 g • Agar 0.3 g • Bromothymol blue (1% aq solution) 0.3 ml • Distilled water 100 ml • Required carbohydrate 1 g	1. Weigh the ingredients. 2. Dissolve the ingredients in a small volume of water. 3. Make up the volume of the medium to 100 ml. 4. Adjust the pH to 7.2. 5. Filter the medium. 6. Distribute in tubes in 5 ml amounts. 7. Sterilize by autoclaving at 8 lbs pressure for 30 minutes. 8. Store at 4°C.

Quality Control

- Check the sterility of the prepared medium by incubating one sample tube at 37°C overnight. No growth indicates sterility of the medium.
- Check the ingredients by inoculating two tubes with known organisms responsible for oxidative and fermentative utilization of carbohydrate. There

should be good growth and change in colour in the whole media in case of fermentative utilization and only on the surface in case of oxidative utilization.

16.7.2.10 Phenylalanine Deaminase Agar

Use: It is used to differentiate members of the genera *Proteus, Morganella* (which were originally classified under the genus *Proteus*), and *Providencia* from other Enterobacteriaceae.

Ingredient	Method of preparation
• Yeast extract 3 g • L -phenylalanine 1 g or DL-phenylalanine 2 g • Disodium hydrogen phosphate 1 g • Sodium chloride 5 g • Agar 12 g • Distilled water 1 litre	1. Weigh the ingredients. 2. Dissolve the ingredients in water by gentle heating. 3. Make up the volume of the medium to 1 litre. 4. Adjust the pH to 7.3. 5. Add agar agar. Dissolve the agar by free steaming or by continuous stirring by placing the container in a water bath. 6. Filter through layers of gauge piece. 7. Distribute in tubes. 8. Sterilize by autoclaving at 15 lbs pressure for 15 minutes. 9. Incline tubes to make long slants. 10. Store at 4°C.

16.7.2.11 Müller-Hinton Agar

Use: It is commonly used for antibiotic susceptibility testing.

Ingredient	Method of preparation
• Beef, dehydrated infusion from 300 g • Casein hydrolysate 17.5 g • Starch 1.5 g • Agar 17 g • Distilled water 1 litre Five percent sheep blood may also be added when susceptibility testing is done on *Streptococcus* species	1. Weigh the ingredients. 2. Dissolve the ingredients in water completely by boiling. 3. Make up the volume of the medium to 1 litre. 4. Adjust the pH to 7.3. 5. Add agar-agar. Dissolve the agar by free steaming or by continuous stirring by placing the container in a water bath. 6. Filter through layers of gauge piece. 7. Sterilize by autoclaving at 121°C for 15 minutes. 8. Cool to 52°C. 9. Pour plates.

16.8 LABORATORY RECORD

Make a record of various culture media prepared by you in the following format.

Date	Name of the medium prepared	Conditions maintained for complete medium				Teacher's signature
		pH	Sterilization condition		Quality control results on control media	
			Before distribution	After distribution		

Cultivation of Bacteria

17.1 AIM

To explain to students different methods of cultivation of organisms, relative importance of cultivating organisms in liquid medium (broth) or in solid medium (agar medium) and methods for agar plate cultures.

17.2 LEARNING OUTCOME

After this exercise, the students
- Shall understand various terms and steps related to cultivation of bacteria.
- Know the purpose of distribution of the culture media in tubes as broth, agar stab and agar slants and in plates as agar plates, etc.
- Attain the required skill for inoculating the materials in liquid medium and in/on the solid medium.
- Know the conditions for incubation of the inoculated media.

17.3 RELATIVE ADVANTAGES AND DISADVANTAGES OF BROTH CULTURE AND AGAR CULTURE

17.3.1 Advantages of using Liquid Medium (Broth) for Cultivation of Bacteria

- For rapid growth of the organisms.
- For performing hanging drop experiment to see the motility.
- For performing biochemical tests.
- For total counting of the organisms.
- For as inoculum for antibiotic sensitivity tests.
- For assessing minimum inhibitory concentration (MIC) of an agent in a broth culture.

Disadvantage

Organisms cannot be isolated in pure culture from a mixed growth.

17.3.2 Advantages of Agar Slant Cultures

Agar slopes/slants are prepared by distributing the agar medium in test tubes/bottles and placing them in a slanting position for solidification. Agar slants are used for:
- Better growth of aerobic organisms
- For performing biochemical tests on pure culture

17.3.3 Advantages of Agar Stab Cultures

Agar stabs are prepared by distributing the agar medium in tubes/small bottles and placing them vertically for solidification. Agar stabs are used for:

- Growth of anaerobic organisms.
- Preservation of bacterial culture.
- For performing certain biochemical tests.
- Seeing motility (in semi-solid stabs).

17.3.4 Advantages of Agar Plate Cultures

Advantages

- Isolation of individual colony from the mixed growth on an agar plate for obtaining pure culture.
- Preliminary identification of the organisms based on the overall growth characteristics and individual colony characteristics.
- Counting of number of living cells (viable counting).
- Putting up of antibiotic sensitivity test.

17.4 CULTIVATION OF ORGANISMS

Cultivation of organisms on artificial medium involves two steps

1. Inoculation in/on medium distributed in tubes as broth, stab, slope/slant or on petridishes.
2. Incubation under desirable growth conditions.

17.4.1 Inoculation

17.4.1(a) Inoculation in Liquid Medium/Broth

- Inoculum transferred from a liquid medium
- Inoculum transferred from an agar medium.

17.4.1(b) Inoculation in Agar Media in Tubes as Agar Stab or Agar Slant and Inoculation on Agar Plates

- Inoculum transferred from a liquid medium
- Inoculum transferred from an agar medium.

17.4.1(c) Inoculum Transferred from a Liquid Medium

- Heat the entire length of the loop to redness before using it to inoculate the broth. This prevents any bacteria from being transferred from the stem of the loop to the broth.
- Cool the loop (by keeping it near the flame) before inserting it in the culture from which the growth is to be transferred.
- Open the tube/bottle containing the broth culture from which transfer is to be made. Use your little and ring finger to hold the cotton wool plugs/caps. Never place the cap or the cotton wool plug on the work bench.
- Flame the rim of the culture tube/bottle after opening.
- Carefully insert the loop into the tube/bottle of broth culture without touching the sides of the tube and pick up a loopful of growth.
- Remove the loop with the culture from the tube/bottle without touching the sides.
- Flame the rim of the culture tube/bottle and close the culture tube/bottle with the plug/cap held between your fingers. Maintain sterility of the plug/cap.
- Open the tube/bottle with fresh medium in which the culture is to be transferred. Keep the plug/cap of this tube between your fingers. Flame the rim of this tube/bottle.

- Dislodge the inoculum in the fresh medium with gentle shaking without touching the glass.
- Flame the rim of the tube and cap it or plug it.
- Sterilize the inoculating loop and place it on its stand (Figs 17.1 A to F).

Transfer of inoculum from a solid (agar) medium to a liquid medium (broth)

- Take the inoculum with a sterile, well cooled inoculating loop following all aseptic precautions
- Dislodge in the fresh liquid medium by gently touching the surface of the liquid (Fig. 17.2(A)).

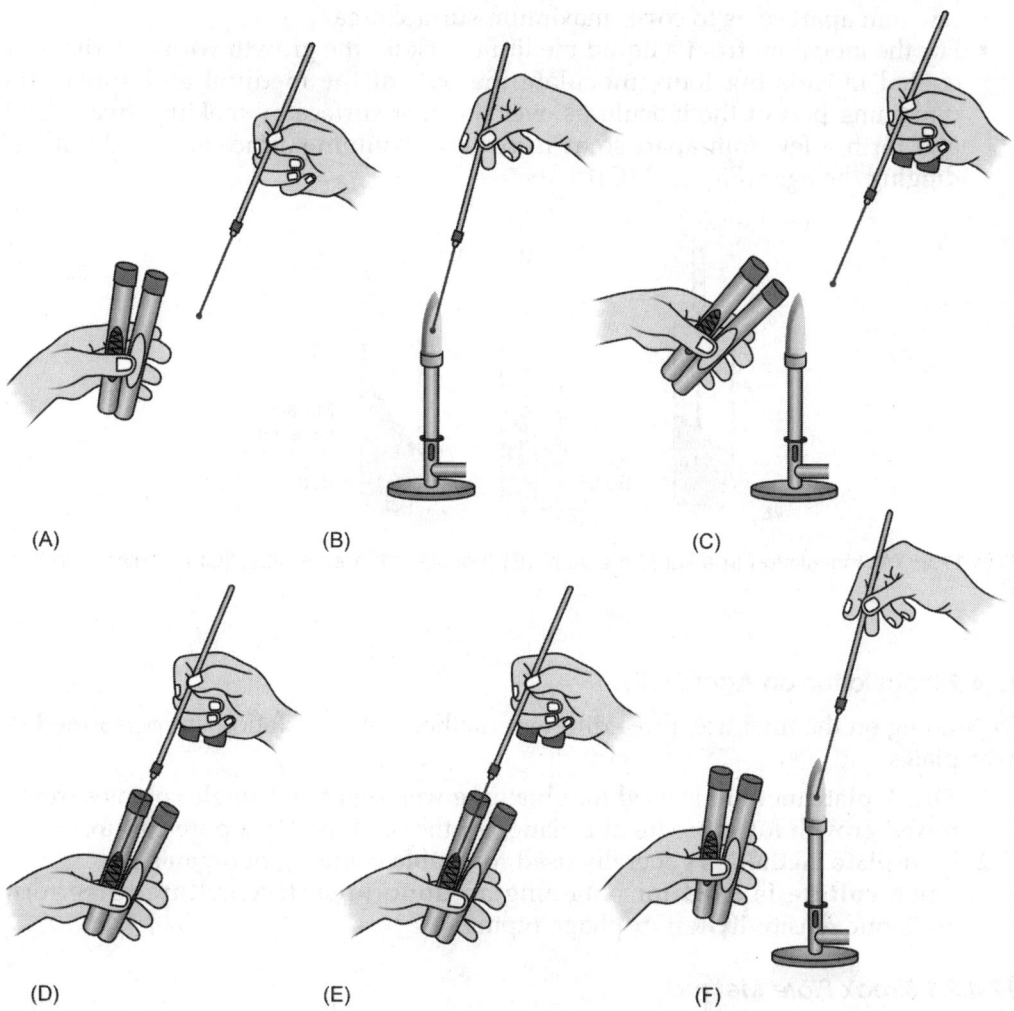

(A)　　　　　　　　(B)　　　　　　　　(C)

(D)　　　　　　　　(E)　　　　　　　　(F)

Figs 17.1 (A to F): Transfer of an inoculum from a culture to a fresh medium (A) Make ready the tubes for transferring the organisms; (B) Sterilize the loop and cool it by holding it close to the flame; (C) Open the caps of th e tubes and hold them between your fingers. Flame the mouth of the tubes; (D) Pick up the growth from one tube with the sterile, cooled loop; (E) Transfer the growth to the tube with fresh medium. Replace the caps; (F) Sterilize the loop again before placing it in the loop holder.

Transfer of Inoculum in Agar Slants and Agar Stabs

Inoculation in agar stabs

- For an inoculum from a solid medium, pick up the growth with a sterile, well cooled straight wire, stab the wire at the bottom of the tube/bottle and slowly work upwards.
- For the inoculum from a liquid medium, pick up the growth with a sterile, well cooled inoculating loop, force the material at the bottom of the tube/bottle and slowly work upwards (Fig. 17.2 (B)).

Inoculation in agar slants/slopes

- For an inoculum from a solid medium, pick up the growth with a sterile, well cooled straight wire, inoculate the butt of the medium and spread the remaining part of the inoculum over the agar surface by making streaks back and forth a few mm apart so as to cover maximum surface area.
- For the inoculum from a liquid medium, pick up the growth with a sterile, well cooled inoculating loop, inoculate the butt of the medium and spread the remaining part of the inoculums over the agar surface by making streaks back and forth a few mm apart so as to cover maximum surface area and without digging the agar (Fig. 17.2 (C)).

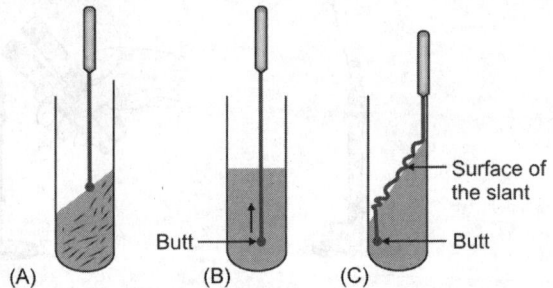

Figs 17.2: (A) Inoculation in a liquid medium, (B) Inoculation in agar stab, (C) Inoculation in agar slant

17.4.2 Inoculation on Agar Plates

Depending on the final use, three different methods of inoculation are performed on agar plates

1. **Streak plate method** is used for obtaining well separated single colonies from a mixed growth for subsequent isolation of the organism in a pure culture.
2. **Pour plate method is** generally used for viable counting of organisms.
3. **Lawn culture is used** for obtaining an uniform surface culture to perform antibiotic sensitivity test or phage typing.

17.4.2.1 Streak Plate Method

1. Take a sterile agar place and dry the surface by keeping the plate upside down on the lid of the petridish.
2. Pick up the inoculum with a sterile, well cooled loop and place it at one upper end of the petridish. Spread the inoculum in the form of a thin smear (base). Streak from the base from side to side in parallel lines to cover approximately one quarter of the plate.

3. Rotate the petridish, flame the inoculating loop, cool and make a second set of streaks from the surface of the first set of streaks.
4. Rotate the petridish once again, flame the inoculating loop, cool and make a third set of streaks from the second set.
5. Close the lid of the plate (Fig. 17.3).

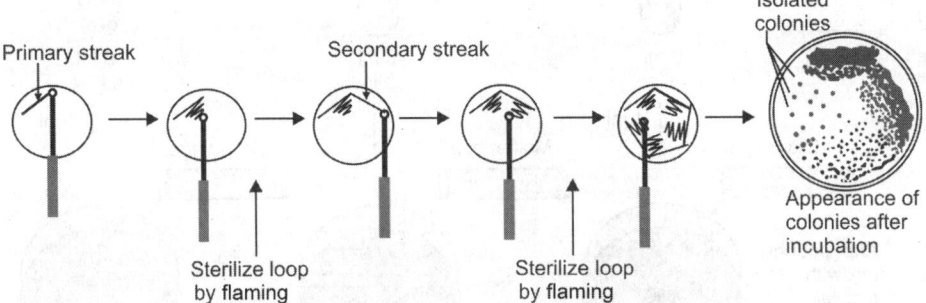

Fig. 17.3: Inoculation by streak plate method

While making streaks, take care that the last set of streaks do not touch the base, streaks cover maximum surface area and the streaks do not touch the periphery of the agar medium.

Pour Plate Method

1. Take sterile petridishes without culture medium.
2. Make tenfold serial dilution of bacterial growth in 9 ml of sterile water or sterile saline or sterile broth as shown in Fig. 17.4.
3. Melt 9 ml of agar medium in tubes by keeping them in water bath.
4. Cool the molten agar media in the tubes to approximately 50°C, mix with 1 ml of the inoculum from each tube using separate sterile pipettes, shake the contents and immediately pour into sterile petridishes. Alternate method is to add 1 ml of the diluted culture to the warm medium already poured in the petridishes mixing with a rotatory movement.
5. Rotate the petridishes gently to distribute the agar uniformly.
6. Allow the agar to set on a leveled surface (Fig. 17.4).

Lawn Culture

Lawn culture is obtaind by spreading or by pouring the inoculum on the agar plate (Fig. 17.5).

(i) Spread plate method

1. Take a sterile agar plate.
2. Soak a sterile swab/spreader in the liquid inoculum.
3. Spread the inoculum with a sterile spreader evenly on the entire agar surface without touching the rim.
4. Dry the surface of the petridish by placing it upside down on the slightly open lid.
5. Close the lid.

(ii) Pour plate method

1. Take sterile agar plate.
2. Pour the broth culture of the organism on the plate.
3. Tilt the plate to cover the surface completely with the liquid inoculum.

1 ml
1 ml
1 ml
Tube 1
10^{-1}
Tube 2
10^{-2}
Tube 3
10^{-3}
Mixed broth culture
9 ml saline
9 ml saline
9 ml saline
1 ml
1 ml
1 ml
Molten agar
Molten agar
Molten agar
After pouring mix with circular motion.
Colony growth after incubation.
Plate 1 (10^{-1}) count the number of colonies
Plate 2 (10^{-2}) count the number of colonies
Plate 3 (10^{-3}) count the number of colonies

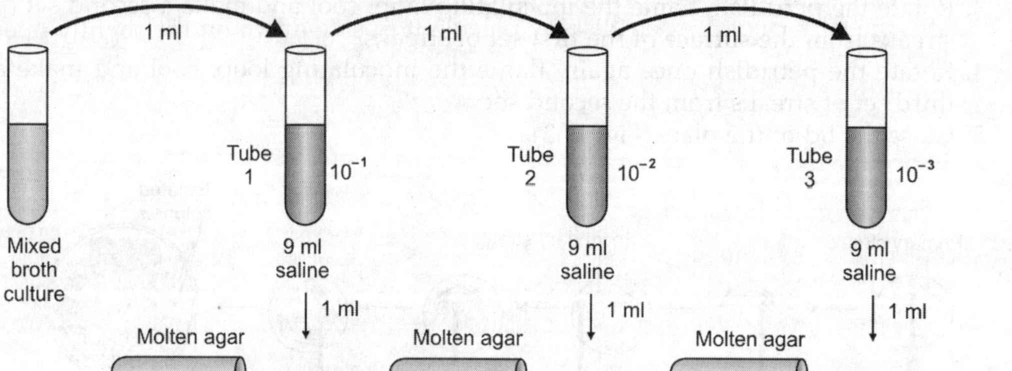

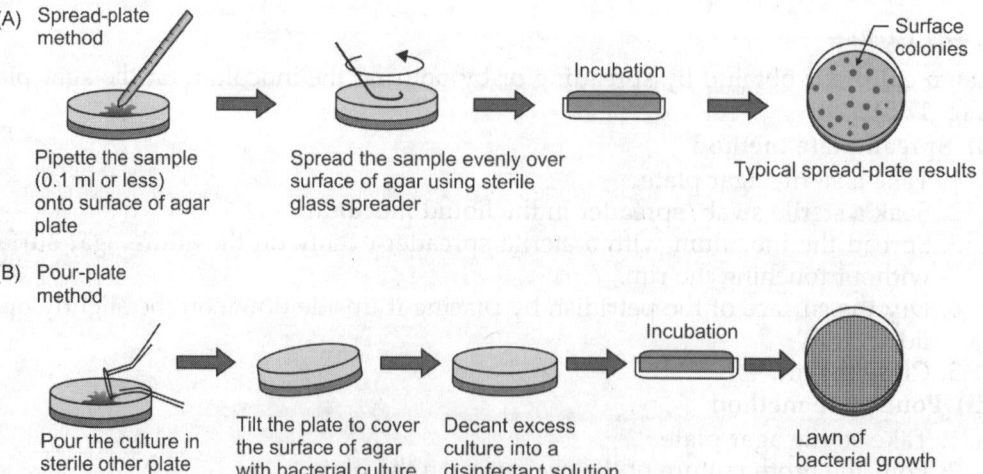

Fig. 17.4: Inoculation by pour plate method

(A) Spread-plate method
Pipette the sample (0.1 ml or less) onto surface of agar plate
Spread the sample evenly over surface of agar using sterile glass spreader
Incubation
Surface colonies
Typical spread-plate results
(B) Pour-plate method
Pour the culture in sterile other plate
Tilt the plate to cover the surface of agar with bacterial culture
Decant excess culture into a disinfectant solution
Incubation
Lawn of bacterial growth

Fig. 17.5: Lawn culture by (A) surface swabbing spread plate method and (B) by pour plate methods

4. Decant excess broth in a disinfecting liquid.
5. Dry the surface of the petridish by placing it upside down on the slightly open lid.
6. Close the lid.

17.5. INCUBATION

17.5.1 For Aerobic Organisms

Keep the inoculated tubes/bottles/plates in the incubator at 37°C for overnight.

17.5.2 For Organisms Requiring Carbon Dioxide Atmosphere

Place the inoculated material in a container (candle jar), lit a candle inside the candle jar, apply grease between lid and rim of the jar and close the container. Burning of the candle shall produce desired carbon dioxide level inside the jar (Fig. 17.6).

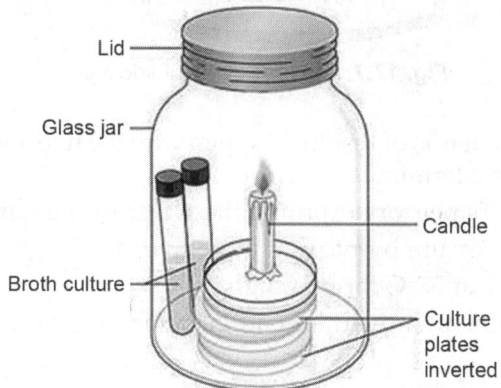

Fig. 17.6: Candle jar

17.5.3 For Anaerobic Organisms

Use a MacIntosh and Filde's jar or a gas pak system.

MacIntosh and Filde's Jar

Construction of the jar: MacIntosh and Filde's jar is a heavy duty jar with flat bottom. The lid of the jar contains two electrical terminals connected with a catalyst comprising of palladium coated asbestos. It also has two tubes for removing the air and for flowing hydrogen inside. There is a gasket to keep the jar air tight (Fig. 17.7).

Principle of working: Anaerobiosis in the MacIntosh jar is created by removal of oxygen through combination of hydrogen in presence of the palladianized asbestos catalyst heated by passing electricity. A tube of methylene blue is kept inside to monitor the anaerobic condition. As long as anaerobic condition is maintained in the jar, methylene blue shall remain colourless.

Procedure

1. Keep the inoculated materials and the methylene blue tube in the jar.
2. Close the jar.
3. With a vacuum pump, remove as much air as possible from inside the jar.
4. Introduce hydrogen gas by connecting the jar with a hydrogen gas producing system.

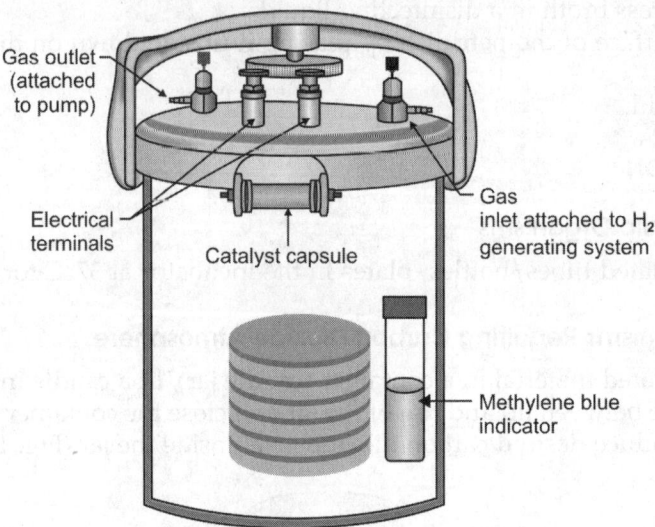

Fig. 17.7: MacIntosh and Filde's jar

5. Catalyze the combination of residual oxygen with the hydrogen by passing current through the electric terminals.
6. Use a sterile filter paper for absorbing the water formed, if any.
7. Restore internal pressure by passing more hydrogen.
8. Keep the assembly at 37°C for overnight.
9. Take out the culture after overnight and examine the growth.

Gas Pak System

Gas pak system uses different chemicals to produce hydrogen and carbon dioxide. It has palladium pellet hanging from the lid to catalyse the combination of hydrogen and oxygen (Fig. 17.8).

For incubation under anaerobic condition, hydrogen is produced by adding water to sodium borohydride in presence of cobalt chloride as catalyst.

$$NaBH_4 + H_2O + \text{cobalt chloride catalyst} \rightarrow NaBO_2 + 4H_2$$

This hydrogen then binds with the oxygen in presence of palladium catalyst to form water.

$$2H_2 + O_2 + \text{palladium catalyst} \rightarrow 2H_2O.$$

For incubation under carbon dioxide atmosphere, pellets of citric acid and sodium bicarbonate are used to produce CO_2.

$$C_3H_5(COOH)_3 + 3NaHCO_3 \rightarrow C_3H_5(COONa)_3 + 3CO_2 + 3H_2O.$$

The disposable envelop contains the required chemicals for carbon dioxide or hydrogen gas production.

Procedure

1. Keep the inoculated plates inside the chamber.
2. Add water to the respective envelops for generation of hydrogen or carbon dioxide.
3. Close the chamber.
4. Incubate at 37°C. Monitor the methylene blue tube for any colour change.

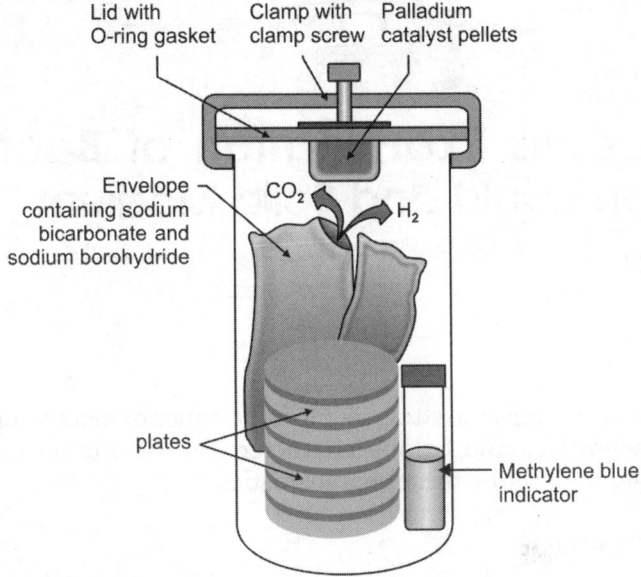

Fig. 17.8: Gas pak system

17.6 LABORATORY RECORD

Maintain a record of cultivation methods performed by you as follows:

Date	Cultivation method performed				Incubation condition			Teacher's signature
	Broth culture	Agar stab	Agar slant	Agar plate	Aerobic	Anaerobic	Carban dioxide	

Macroscopic Examination of Bacterial Growth on Liquid and Solid Medium

18.1 AIM

To create awareness amongst the students the importance of macroscopic examination of growth characteristics and colony characteristics of microorganisms and the terminologies used to describe these characteristics.

18.2 LEARNING OUTCOME

The students can independently examine the growth characteristics of organisms in liquid medium and colony characteristics on agar medium with appropriate description leading to preliminary identification of the organisms.

18.3 GENERAL GROWTH CHARACTER OF ORGANISMS IN BROTH CULTURE

Examine the growth character of the organism in the broth culture at the surface of the liquid and in the body of the liquid.

18.3.1 At the Surface of the Liquid

Examine for
- Ring formation
- Pellicle formation
- Membrane formation.

18.3.2. In the Body of the Liquid

Examine for
- Uniform turbidity.
- Flocculi in suspension.
- Granules in suspension.
- Presence of precipitate or sediment at the bottom of tube with a clear supernatant.
- Presence or absence of colouration of fluid (Fig. 18.1).

18.4 GENERAL GROWTH CHARACTER OF BACTERIA IN STAB CULTURE

Stab Culture

Examine the growth character of the organism in the stab culture along line of puncture and also for liquefaction, if any.

Type of growth along line of puncture: (Fig. 18.2)

a. Filiform: Uniform growth filling the line of inoculation.

b. Echinate: Has pointed processes grown laterally along the line of inoculation.

c. Beaded: Consists of loosely placed colonies resembling beads.

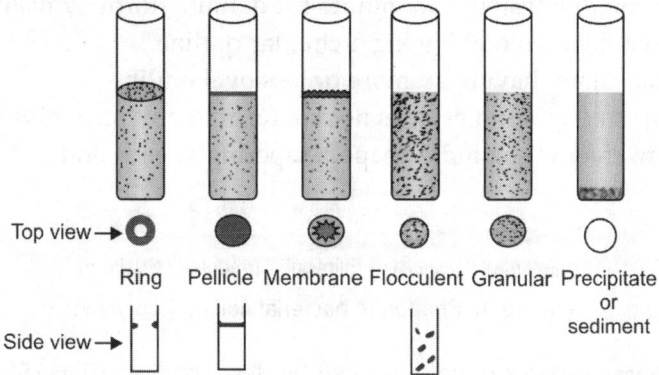

Fig. 18.1: Growth characteristics of organisms in a broth culture

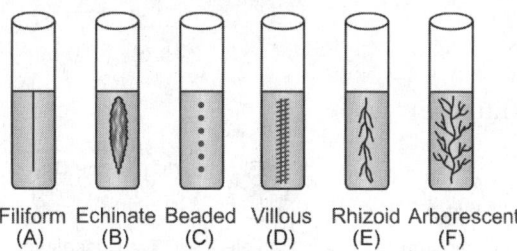

Fig. 18.2: Growth character in agar stab

d. Villous: Has short, undivided, hair-like projections on line of inoculation.

e. Rhizoid: Growth like roots of plants.

f. Arborescent: Branched or tree-like, having branched extensions.

Bulk growth at the surface of the medium indicates that organisms grown are aerobic and bulk growth in the depth of the broth or stab indicates that the organisms are anaerobic.

18.5 PLATE CULTURE

18.5.1 Report General Growth Character (Depending on the Medium used) as under

- On blood agar plate, presence or absence of hemolysis and swarming. Haemolysis, if present, may be complete hemolysis (β-hemolysis) or incomplete haemolysis (α hemolysis) with greenish discolouration.

- On MacConkey or deoxycholate citrate agar media, presence or absence of lactose fermenting colonies.

- On nutrient agar, presence or absence of pigments. Pigments may be soluble or insoluble. Swarming growth may be seen on a nutrient agar medium with less agar.

18.5.2 Colony Characteristics

Distinguish superficial from deep colonies, note the characters of the individual colonies and report the following:

a. Size the diameter in millimeters, after a specific duration of incubation.

b. Shape/form/plan (view from the top) (*see* in Fig. 18.3)

- Punctiform: dimensions too minute for defining form by naked eye.
- Round/circular: colony having a circular outline.
- Elliptical: colony having an more or less oval outline.
- Irregular: colony outlines does not conform to any recognised shape.
- Fusiform: colony is spindle-shaped, tapering at each end.

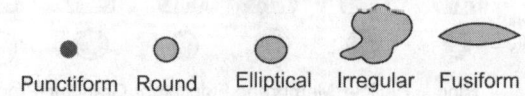

Punctiform Round Elliptical Irregular Fusiform

Fig. 18.3: Shapes of bacterial colony (top view)

c. **Surface characteristics** of colonies can be described as: (Fig. 18.4)
- Smooth
- Contoured
- Radiate
- Concentric
- Wrinkled/(Rugose)

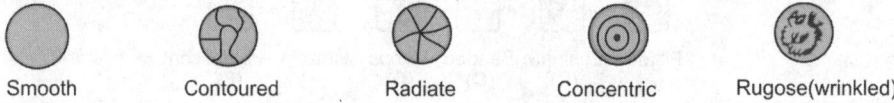

Smooth   Contoured   Radiate   Concentric   Rugose(wrinkled)

Fig. 18.4: Surface characteristics of colonies

d. **Elevation characteristics** of colonies are shown in Fig. 18.5 and are described as follows:
- Effused/swarming: spread over the surface as a thin layer.
- Flat: thin, leaf like colony.
- Raised: thick colony, with terraced edges.
- Convex: surface of the colony is like the segment of a circle.
- Pulvinate: surface of the colony is decidedly convex.
- Umbilicate: surface of the colony has a central pit or depression.
- Conical: surface is like a cone with rounded top.
- Umbonate: has a central convex elevation like an umbrella.

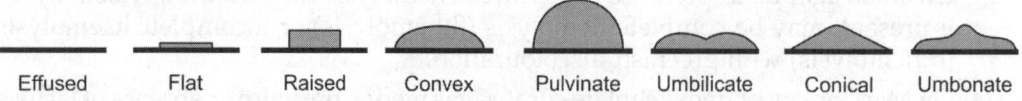

Effused   Flat   Raised   Convex   Pulvinate   Umbilicate   Conical   Umbonate

Fig. 18.5: Surface elevation characteristics of colonies

e. **Margin/edges of colonies** (Fig. 18.6)
- Entire: margin without division.
- Undulate: margin wavy.
- Lobate. margins like lobes.
- Lacerate: margin as if torn.
- Fimbriate: fringed margin.
- Ciliate: margins having hair-like extensions.

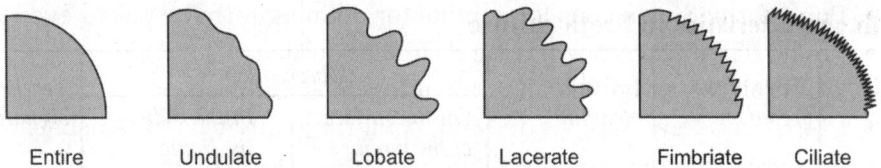

Fig. 18.6: Margin characteristics of colonies

f. Optical characters

Pigment production

1. Describe
   - Colour of pigment.
   - Whether pigment restricted to the colonies (i.e. insoluble pigment).
   - Whether pigment is dispersed in the medium surrounding colonies (i.e. soluble pigment).

2. **Opacity** *general characters*:
   - Transparent: colonies transmits light.
   - Opalescent: colonies translucent; appears as greyish-white when viewed by reflected light.
   - Opaque.
   - Dull/matt: colonies without lustre.
   - Glistening: shining colonies.
   - Fluorescent: colonies reflecting different colour.
   - Mucoid.

18.6 LABORATORY RECORD

1. Inoculate following organisms in nutrient broth, nutrient agar stab, nutrient gelatin stab and on nutrient agar, MacConkey agar and blood agar plates.
   - *Escherichia coli*
   - *Klebsiella* species
   - *Pseudomonas aeruginosa*
   - *Proteus vulgaris*
   - *Staphylococcus aureus*
   - *Streptococcus pyogenes*
   - *Streptococcus viridans*
2. Incubate overnight at 37°C
3. Examine the growth characteristics and record your findings as under:

Growth characteristics in broth culture

Date	Name of the organism	Growth medium	Observation		Teacher's signature
			On the surface of the liquid	In the body of the liquid	

Growth characteristics in stab culture

Date	Name of the organism	Growth medium	Observation		Teacher's signature
			On line of puncture	Type of liquefaction, if any	

Growth characteristics on plate culture

Date	Name of the organism	Growth medium	Overall growth character		Colony characteristics				Teacher's signature
			Pigment production	Optical properties	Size	Type	Elevation	Margin	

19

Study of Biochemical Activities of Bacteria in Culture Medium

19.1 AIM

To study utilization of various nutrients by the bacteria and to detect production of various metabolic end products and enzymes in the culture leading to preliminary identification of the organisms.

19.2 LEARNING OBJECTIVES

After this exercise, the students can carry out the biochemical tests and can detect various metabolic end products in a bacterial culture.

19.3 GENERAL PRINCIPLE

Routine tests for examining the biochemical activities of bacteria are broadly classified as under:

- Tests for metabolic end products in the growth medium.
- Tests for specific enzyme production.

19.3.1 Tests for Metabolic End Products using Specific Media

Utilization of carbohydrate and other energy sources

- Carbohydrate utilization test.
- Methyl red test.
- Voges Proskauer reaction.
- Citrate utilization test.

Utilization of proteins and other nitrogen containing compounds

- Indole test.
- Hydrogen sulphide production test.
- Nitrate reductase test.
- Urease test.
- Phenylalanine deaminase test.
- Gelatin liquefaction test.

19.3.2 Tests for Enzyme Production (No Specific Medium Required)

- Catalase test.
- Coagulase test.
- Oxidase test.

19.3.1.1 (a) Carbohydrate Fermentation Test

Purpose

Carbohydrate fermentation test is done for preliminary identification of bacteria.

Principle

Carbohydrate fermentation test demonstrates the production of acid (with or without gas production) as the metabolic end product of carbohydrate utilization. The acid production is detected by an acid base indicator included in the medium. For detection of the gas production, Durham's tube is added.

Carbohydrate → (glycolysis/fermentation) → pyruvic acid → lactic acid, acetic acid, etc. (depending on the organism) +/− gas production (Fig. 19.1)

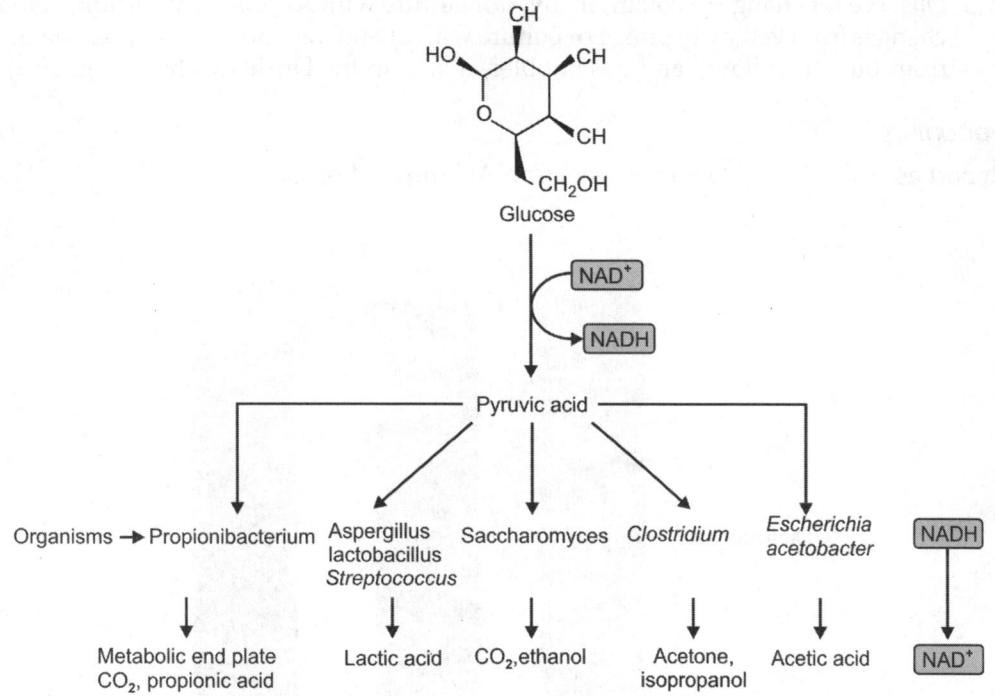

Fig. 19.1: Principle of carbohydrate fermentation test

Materials Required

- Different carbohydrates, viz., glucose, fructose, galactose, sucrose, arabinose, ribose, xylose, maltose, mannitol, etc.
- Peptone water medium.
- 0.5% Andrade's indicator (prepared by adding 1N sodium hydroxide to a 0.5% solution of fuchsin in distilled water until the colour just becomes yellow) or 0.01% phenol red indicator.
- Test tubes 3" × 1/2" and Durham's tube.
- Known bacterial culture (pure cultures of *Escherichia coli*, *Staphylococcus aureus* and other organisms.

Preparation of the Carbohydrate Fermentation Test Medium

1. Add 1g of each carbohydrate in 100 ml of peptone water medium placed in different conical flasks.
2. Add 1 ml of 0.5% Andrade's indicator or 0.1 ml of 0.01% phenol red indicator in each of the flasks.
3. Distribute in 3" × 1/2" tubes. Invert Durham's tube in each tube.
4. Colour the top of the cotton plugs on the tubes according to the standard colour code for each sugar.
5. Keep in racks.
6. Sterilize at 8 lbs pressure for 30 minutes.

Procedure

1. Inoculate known bacteria in the sugar set.
2. Incubate overnight at 37°C.
3. Observe for change in colour, if any, (for culture with Andrade's indicator, colour changes from yellow to pink. For culture with phenol red indicator, colour changes from pink to yellow), and gas bubbles, if any, in the Durham's tube (Fig. 19.2).

Reporting

Report as A (acid), AG (acid and gas) or NAG (no acid or gas)

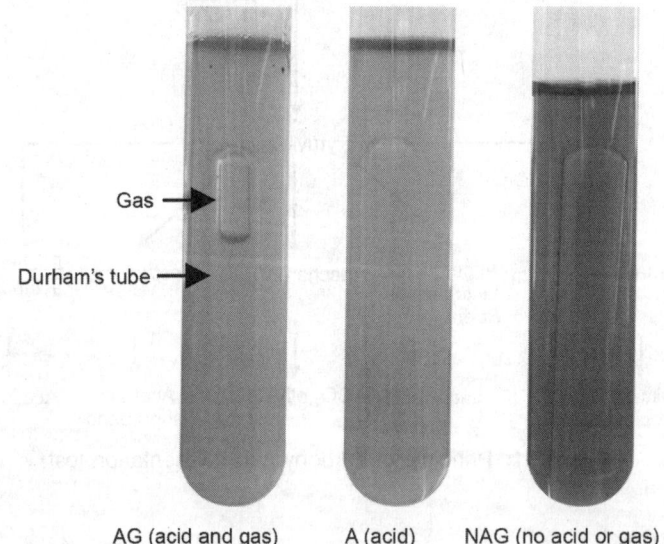

Fig. 19.2: Carbohydrate fermentation test (*see* colour plate 3)

19.3.1.1 (a) Demonstration of Oxidative–fermentative Utilization of Carbohydrates

Purpose

Oxidative-fermentative test determines if certain Gram-negative rods metabolize carbohydrate by fermentation (anaerobic utilization) or by aerobic respiration (oxidative utilization). Two tubes of Hugh-Leifson media are taken for inoculating each carbohydrate and after inoculation one tube is covered with a layer of paraffin oil.

Principle

During the anaerobic process of **fermentation, pyruvate is converted to a variety of mixed acids in high concentration** depending on the type of bacteria carrying out **the fermentation** turning the bromothymol blue indicator **green to yellow in both open and paraffin layered tubes**.

Glucose → pyruvic acid → lactic acid/acetic acid, etc. (depending on the organism) (Fig. 19.1)

Certain oxidative bacteria **metabolize glucose using aerobic respiration** and therefore **only produce a small amount of weak acids,** mostly oxaloacetic acid and succinic acid **(pH 6.0)** during the Krebs cycle (Fig. 19.3). After 24 hours incubation, a **change in the colour of the bromothymol blue indicator is observed only at the surface of the open tube** where growth in presence of oxygen is observed (Fig. 19.4).

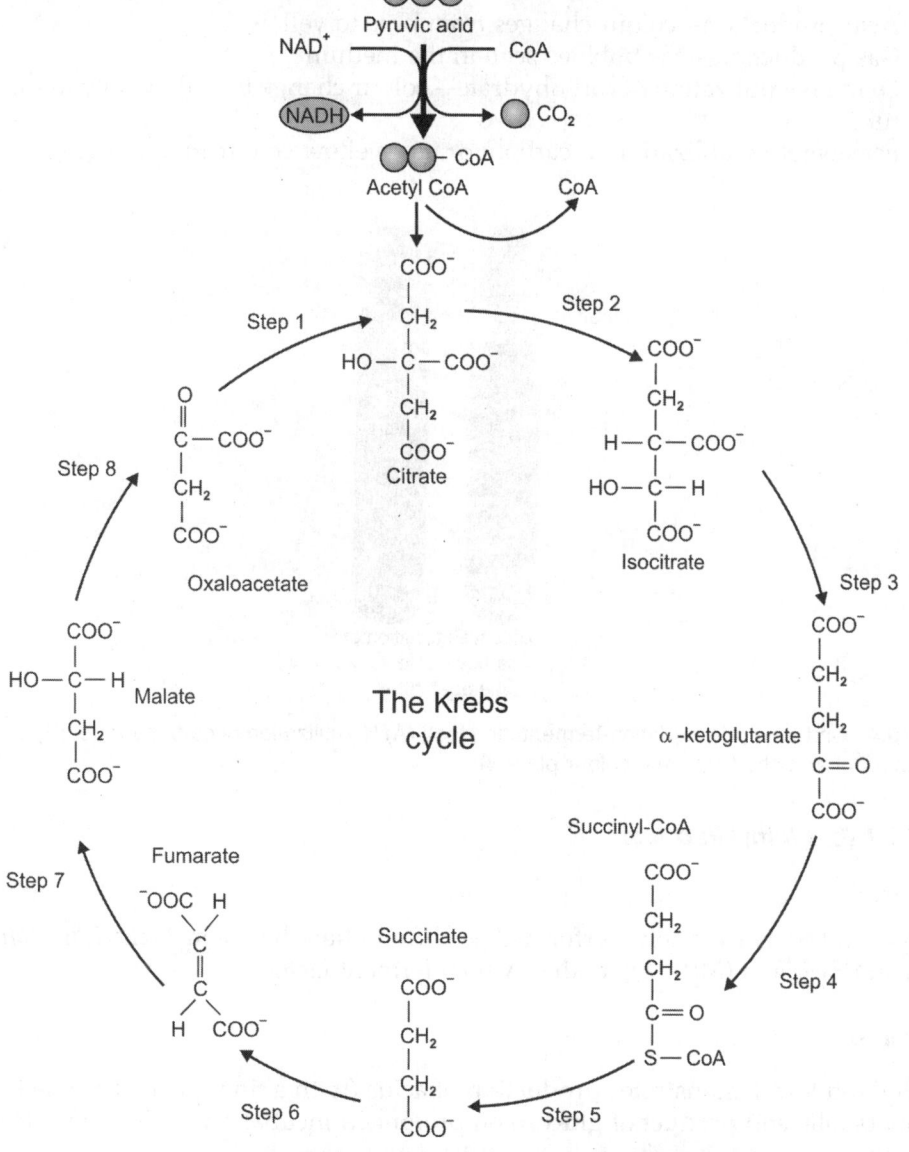

Fig. 19.3: Principle of oxidative utilization of carbohydrates

Hugh-Leifson media shall not change the colour if non-saccharolytic bacteria is inoculated.

Materials Required

- Hugh and Leifson's agar stab with different carbohydrates.
- Pure culture of known bacteria, *Escherichia coli*, and *Pseudomonas*, etc.
- Sterile paraffin.

Procedure

1. Stab inoculate two tubes of each carbohydrate with the bacteria.
2. Cover one tube with a layer of sterile paraffin.
3. Incubate at 37°C for up to 14 days.

Observation

- Acid production—colour changes from blue to yellow.
- Gas production—gas bubbles seen in the medium.
- Oxidative utilization of carbohydrate—colour change to yellow only in the open tube.
- Fermentative utilization of carbohydrate—yellow colour in both tubes.

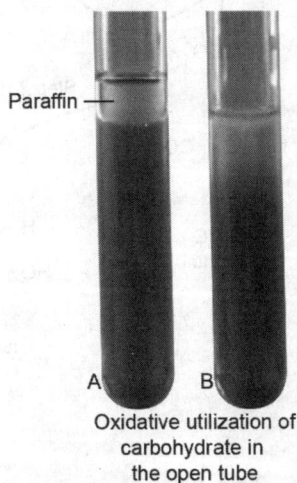

Paraffin

A   B

Oxidative utilization of
carbohydrate in
the open tube

Fig. 19.4: Carbohydrate oxidation-fermentation test: (A) No utilization of carbohydrate, (B) oxidative utilization of carbohydrate (*see* colour plate 3)

19.3.1.1 (b) Methyl Red Test

Purpose

Metyl red test is routinely performed to differentiate between *Escherichia coli* (MR +ve) and *Klebsiella* (MR –ve), both of which ferment lactose.

Principle

Methyl red test demonstrates production of acids (with a final pH of 4.5 or below) as the metabolic end product of glucose on prolonged incubation of certain bacteria for 48 hours.

Glucose + H_2O—> lactic acid/acetic acid/formic acid, (pH < 4.5 depending on the species of bacteria, changing the methyl red colour to red) +CO_2 (Fig. 19.5)

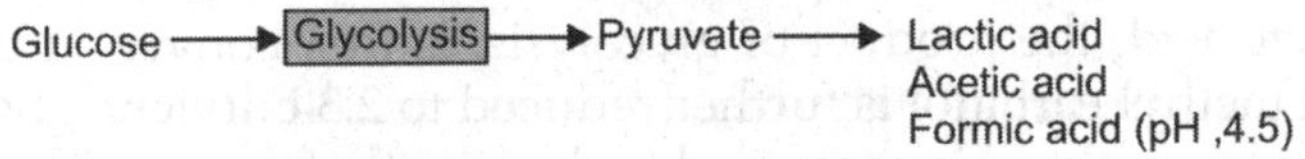

Glucose ⟶ Glycolysis ⟶ Pyruvate ⟶ Lactic acid
                                                                    Acetic acid
                                                                    Formic acid (pH ,4.5)

Fig. 19.5: Principle of methyl red test

Materials Required

- Pure culture of *Escherichia coli* and *Klebsiella*.
- Sterile glucose phosphate peptone water medium distributed in small tubes.
- Methyl red solution (0.1g of methyl red in 300 ml ethanol and 200 ml distilled water).

Procedure

1. Inoculate the bacteria in glucose phosphate peptone water medium.
2. Incubate at 37°C for 48 hours.
3. Add 5 drops of methyl red to this old culture.
4. Observe immediately.

Observation

- Positive test-bright red colour of methyl red
- Negative test-yellow (Fig. 19.6).

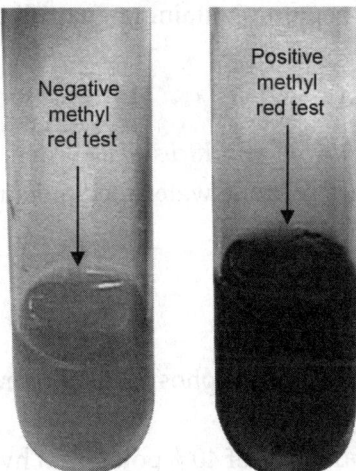

Negative methyl red test

Positive methyl red test

Fig. 19.6: Demonstration of methyl red test (*see* colour plate 3)

19.3.1.1 (c) Voges-Proskauer (VP) Reaction

Purpose

VP test is done to differentiate between *Escherichia coli* (VP –ve) and *Klebsiella* (VP +ve) both of which ferment lactose.

Principle

Voges-Proskauer test demonstrates production of diacetyl as the end product of glucose metabolism by certain bacteria on prolonged incubation (Fig. 19.7). In this series of reactions, pyruvic acid, the product of glycolysis, is first converted to acetyl methyl carbinol. Acetyl methyl carbinol is further reduced to 2,3 butylene glycol. In presence of KOH, 2,3, butylenes glycol is converted to diacetyl that reacts with α- naphthol and the guanidine groups present in the amino acids (cysteine, arginine, etc. present in peptone) to produce a red colour.

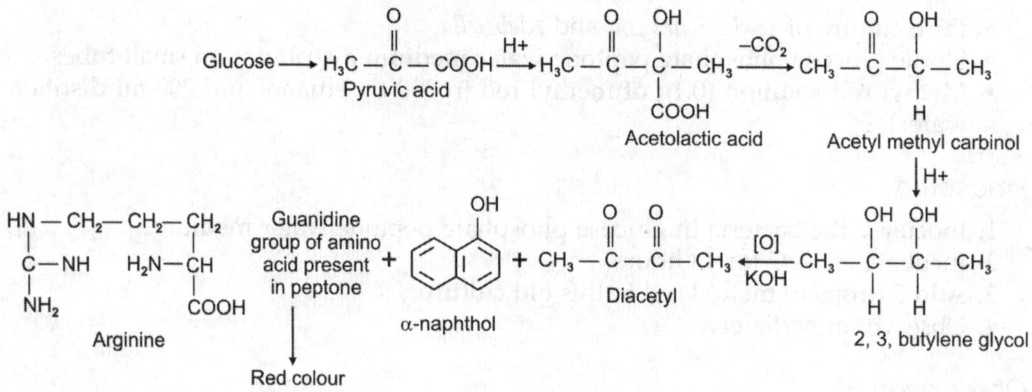

Fig. 19.7: Principle of Voges-Proskauer reaction

Diacetyl + amino acids of peptone containing **guanidine group** (e.g. arginine) + α-naphthol → red colour

Materials Required

- Pure culture of *Escherichia coli* and *Klebsiella*.
- Sterile glucose phosphate peptone water media distributed in tubes.
- 40% potassium hydroxide solution.
- 5% a naphthol in absolute alcohol.

Procedure

1. Inoculate the organism in glucose phosphate peptone water.
2. Incubate at 37 for 48 hours.
3. To 5 ml of the culture, add 1 ml of 40% potassium hydroxide solution and shake well.
4. Add 3 ml of 5% α-naphthol solution.
5. Observe the reaction for 30 minutes.

Observation

- A positive test, i.e. the production of acetyl methyl carbinol is indicated by development of pink colour in 2 to 5 minutes that becomes darker in 30 minutes (Fig. 19.8).

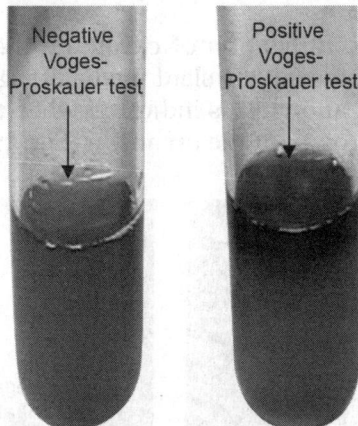

Fig. 19.8: Demonstration of Voges-Proskauer test (*see* colour plate 3)

19.3.1.1 (d) Citrate Utilization Test

Purpose

Citrate utilization test is a routine test to differentiate between *Escherichia coli* (citrate –ve) and *Klebsiella* (citrate +ve).

Principle

Citrate utilization test demonstrates the ability of certain organisms to utilize citrate as sole source of carbon and energy. Citrate is converted by the organism to CO_2 that combines with sodium ion to form sodium carbonate and the pH change is detected by a pH indicator included in the medium (Fig. 19.9).

(a) Sodium citrate → citric acid ($C_6 H_8 O_7$) + Na^+

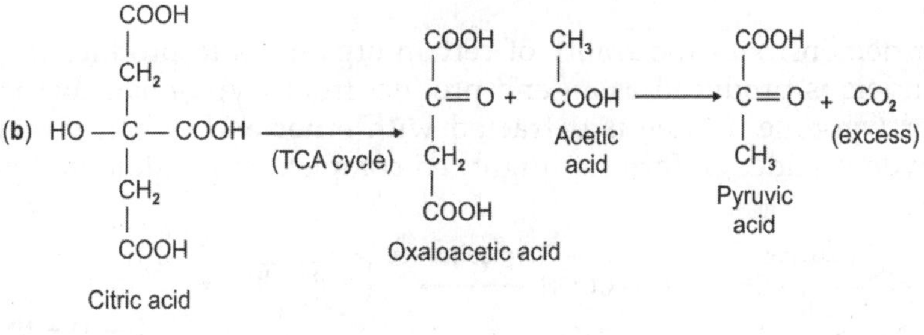

(b)

$$\underset{\text{Citric acid}}{\begin{array}{c} COOH \\ | \\ CH_2 \\ | \\ HO-C-COOH \\ | \\ CH_2 \\ | \\ COOH \end{array}} \xrightarrow{\text{(TCA cycle)}} \underset{\text{Oxaloacetic acid}}{\begin{array}{c} COOH \\ | \\ C=O \\ | \\ CH_2 \\ | \\ COOH \end{array}} + \underset{\substack{\text{Acetic} \\ \text{acid}}}{\begin{array}{c} CH_3 \\ | \\ COOH \end{array}} \longrightarrow \underset{\substack{\text{Pyruvic} \\ \text{acid}}}{\begin{array}{c} COOH \\ | \\ C=O \\ | \\ CH_3 \end{array}} + \underset{\text{(excess)}}{CO_2}$$

(c) $2CO_2 + 2Na^+ + H_2O \longrightarrow Na_2CO_3 \longrightarrow$ Alkaline $\longrightarrow$ Colour of medium
(PH > 7.6)   changes from
green to blue

Fig. 19.9: Principle of citrate utilization test

Materials Required

- Simmon's citrate medium distributed as agar slants.
- Pure cultures of *Escherichia coli* and *Klebsiella*.

Procedure

1. Inoculate citrate agar slants with the bacterial culture.
2. Incubate at 37°C for overnight.
3. Examine for growth and colour change.

Observation

- A positive test, i.e. the utilization of citrate by the organism is indicated by development of blue colour in the slant media along with a streak of growth.
- A negative citrate utilization test is indicated when there is no colour change in the slant and also no growth of the organism (Fig. 19.10).

Positive citrate utilization test

Negative citrate utilization test

Fig. 19.10: Demonstration of citrate utilization test (*see* colour plate 4)

19.3.1.2 Metabolism of Proteins and other Nitrogen Containing Compounds by Bacteria

19.3.1.2 (a) Indole Test

Purpose

Indole test is routinely done to differentiate between *Escherichia coli* (indole + ve) and *Klebsiella* (Indole –ve).

Principle

Indole test demonstrates the ability of certain organisms to produce tryptophanase enzyme. Indole is produced as an end product from tryptophan that is present in peptone or tryptone. Indole is extracted with ether and, when p-methyl amino benzaldehyde is added, it forms a bright red complex with indole in the ether layer (Fig. 19.11).

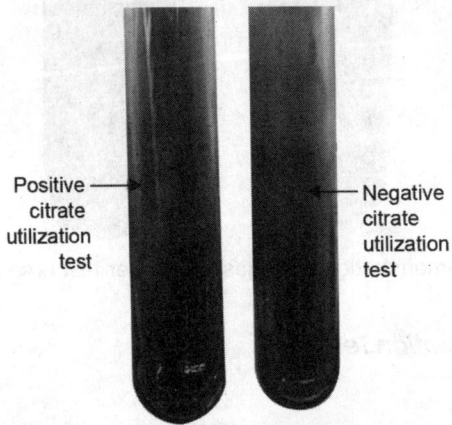

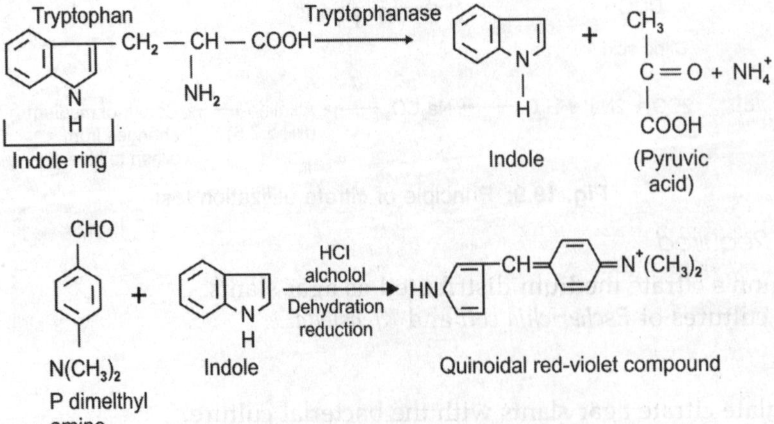

Fig. 19.11: Principle of indole test

Materials Required

- Sterile peptone water or tryptone water medium distributed in tubes.
- Pure culture of *Escherichia coli* and *Klebsiella*.
- Kovac's indole reagent or Ehrlich's indole reagent.
- Ether.

Preparation of Kovac's indole reagent: Dissolve 10 g of paradimethyl aminobenzaldehyde in 150 ml of reagent grade amyl alcohol or isoamyl alcohol. Slowly add 50 ml of conc. pure hydrochloric acid, mix well. Store in the refrigerator in a bottle with proper labeling.

Preparation of Ehrlich indole reagent: Dissolve 1 g of paradimethyl aminobenzaldehyde in 95 ml of absolute ethanol. Slowly add 20 ml of conc pure hydrochloric acid, mix well. Store in the refrigerator in a bottle with proper labeling.

Procedure

1. Inoculate peptone water or tryptone water with the bacteria.
2. Incubate at 37°C for overnight.
3. Shake the culture with approximately 1 ml of ether.
4. Allow the ether layer to stabilize at the top of the culture.
5. Slowly add 0.5 ml of either Kovac's reagent or Ehrlich reagent.
6. Observe the colour in the ether layer.

Observation

A positive test, i.e. indole production by the organism is indicated by development of rose purple colour in the ether layer (Fig. 19.12).

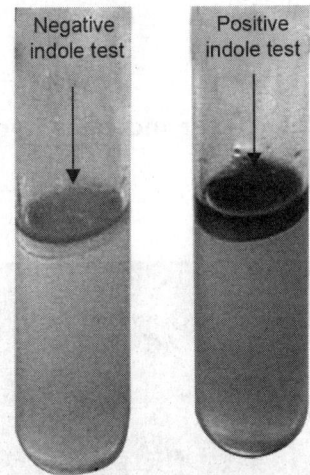

Fig. 19.12: Demonstration of indole test (*see* colour plate 4)

19.3.1.2 (b) Hydrogen Sulphide Production Test

Purpose: Hydrogen sulphide production test is done to differentiate *Escherichia coli* (H_2S +ve) from *Klebsiella* (H_2S –ve) and also *Salmonella* (H_2S +ve) from *Shigella* (H_2S –ve).

Principle

Hydrogen sulphide production test demonstrates the ability of certain organisms to produce hydrogen sulphide from sulphur containing amino acids present in peptone. Hydrogen sulphide is detected by placing a strip coated with saturated lead acetate solution (Fig. 19.13).

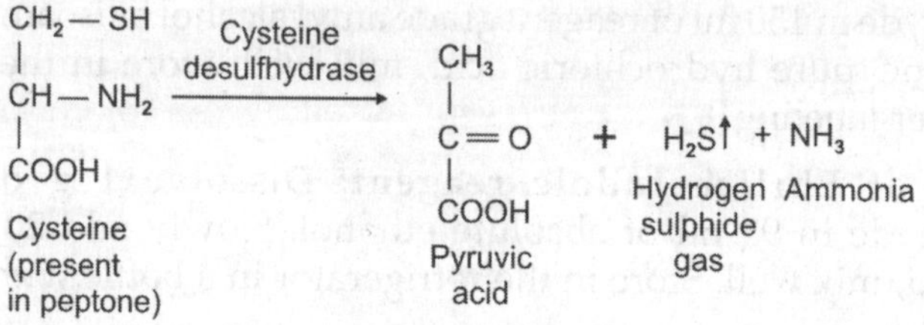

$$CH_2-SH \quad \xrightarrow[\text{desulfhydrase}]{\text{Cysteine}} \quad CH_3$$

$$CH-NH_2 \qquad\qquad\qquad C=O \quad + \quad H_2S\uparrow + NH_3$$

COOH

Cysteine   COOH   Hydrogen Ammonia
(present   Pyruvic   sulphide
in peptone)   acid   gas

$$H_2S + \text{Lead acetate} \longrightarrow \text{PBS (black)}$$

Fig. 19.13: Principle of hydrogen sulphide production test

Materials Required

- Sterile peptone water medium distributed in tubes.
- Pure culture of *Escherichia coli* and *Klebsiella*.
- Filter paper strips soaked in saturated lead acetate solution, dried and sterilized.

Procedure

1. Inoculate peptone water with the bacteria.
2. Place the lead acetate strip in the broth culture.
3. Incubate at 37°C for overnight.
4. Observe the strip for blackening.

Observation

Blackening of the lead acetate paper indicates hydrogen sulphide production (Fig. 19.14).

19.3.1.2 (c) Urease Test

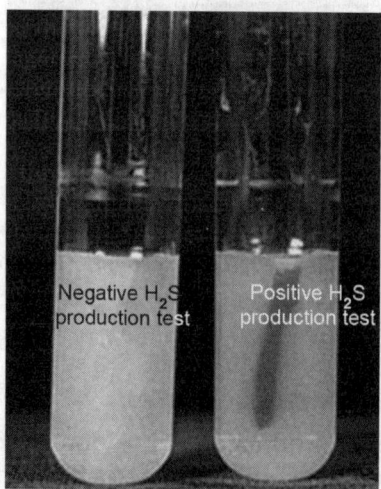

Negative H$_2$S production test   Positive H$_2$S production test

Fig. 19.14: Demonstration of H$_2$S production test (*see* colour plate 4)

Purpose

Urease test is done to confirm *Proteus* and *Klebsiella* which are urease positive (Fig. 19.15).

Principle

Urease test demonstrates the ability of certain organisms to produce urease enzyme that splits urea to ammonia and carbon dioxide. Culture becomes alkaline due to production of ammonia. Change in pH is indicated by the colour change of phenol red indicator (incorporated in the media) to red.

Materials Required

$$\frac{NH_2}{NH_2}\!\!>\!C=O + 2H_2O \xrightarrow{\text{Urease}} CO_2 + 2NH_3 + H_2O$$

Carbon Ammonia Water
dioxide

↓

Turns phenol
red pink

Fig. 19.15: Principle of urease test

- Sterile Christensen's urease medium distributed in slope.
- Pure cultures of *Proteus*, *Escherichia coli* and *Klebsiella*.

Procedure

1. Inoculate the medium with the bacteria.
2. Incubate at 37°C for overnight.
3. Examine the colour change, if any.

Observation

A positive test for urease production is indicated by development of pink colour due to release of ammonia in the medium and subsequent colour change of phenol red indicator (Fig. 19.16).

19.3.1.2 (d) Nitrate Reduction Test

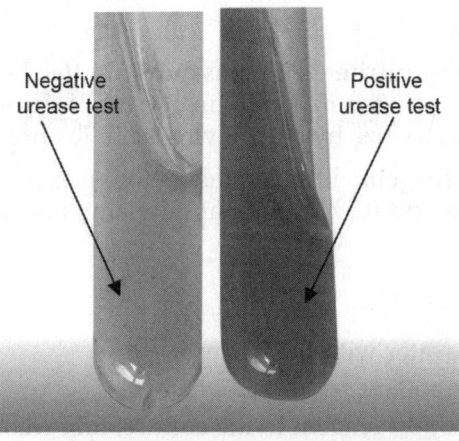

Negative
urease test

Positive
urease test

Fig. 19.16: Demonstration of urease production test (*see* colour plate 4)

Purpose

Nitrate reduction test is useful for separating members of the family Enterobacteriaceae from other Gram-negative bacilli and also for identifying species of *Neisseria* and facilitating species identification of *Corynebacterium*.

Principle

Nitrate reduction is carried out by certain organisms that can produce nitrate reductase enzyme converting nitrate to nitrite. Nitrite is subsequently detected by diazo test (Fig. 19.17).

Materials Required

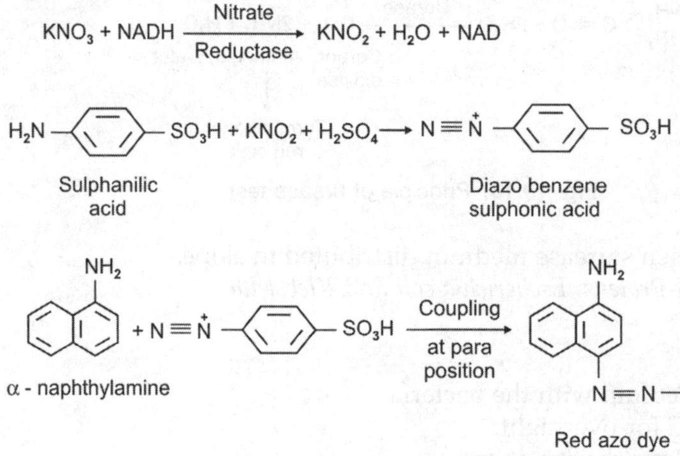

$$KNO_3 + NADH \xrightarrow[\text{Reductase}]{\text{Nitrate}} KNO_2 + H_2O + NAD$$

Fig. 19.17: Principle of nitrate reductase test

- Sterile peptone water medium containing nitrite free potassium nitrate and distributed in tubes.
- Pure culture of *Escherichia coli*, *Klebsiella* and other organisms.
- 0.8% sulphanilic acid in 100 ml of 5 N acetic acid.
- 0.5% alpha naphthylamine in 5 N acetic acid.
- 5 N acetic acid.

Preparation of Materials

Peptone water containing nitrite free potassium nitrate: Dissolve 0.5 g of peptone and 0.02 g of nitrite free potassium nitrate in 100 ml of distilled water, distribute in tubes in 5 ml quantities, sterilize by autoclaving at 15 lbs pressure for 15 minutes.

Preparation of diazo reagent: Immediately before use, mix equal volumes of 0.8% sulphanilic acid solution and 0.5% alpha-naphthylamine solution to make the diazo reagent.

Procedure

1. Inoculate peptone water with the bacteria.
2. Incubate overnight at 37°C.
3. Add 0.1 ml of diazo test reagent to the culture, mix well.
4. Examine the tube for development of a red colour within a few minutes.

Plate 1

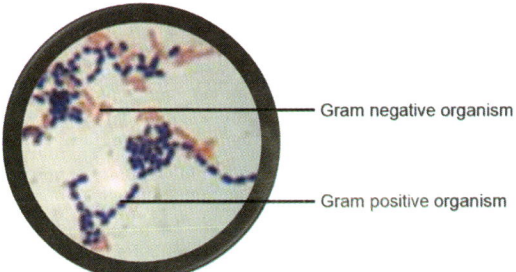

Fig. 12.3: Gram-positive and Gram-negative organisms

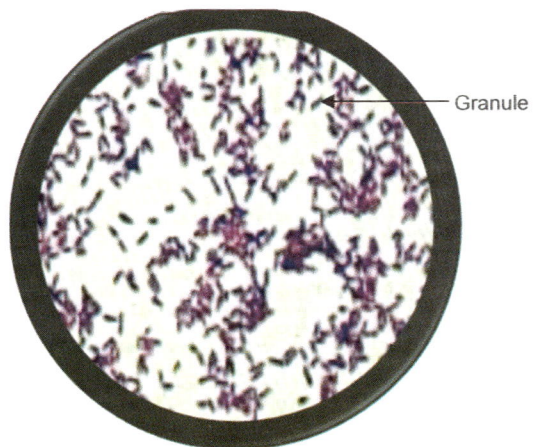

Fig. 12.4: Gram-positive organism (diphtheria bacillus) with granules

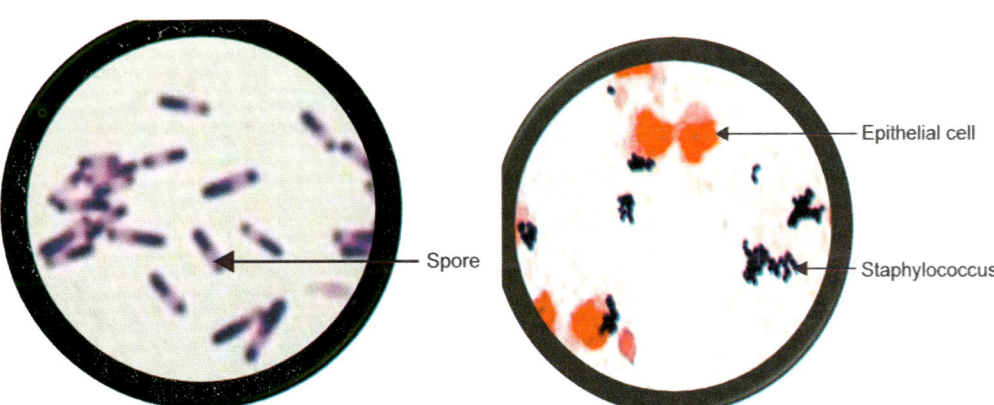

Fig. 12.5: Gram-positive spore bearing organisms (*Clostridium*)   **Fig. 12.6:** *Staphylococcus* in a sputum sample

Plate 2

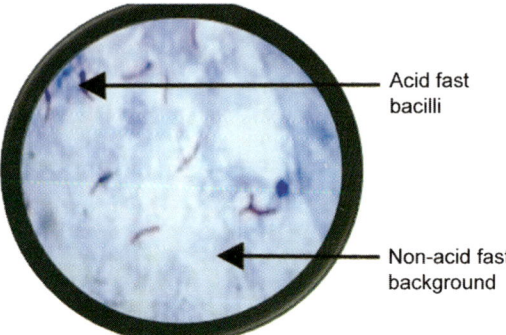

Fig. 13.4: *Mycobacterium tuberculosis*

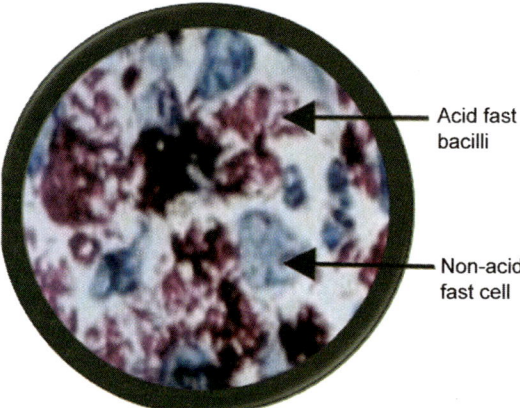

Fig. 13.5: *Mycobacterium leprae*

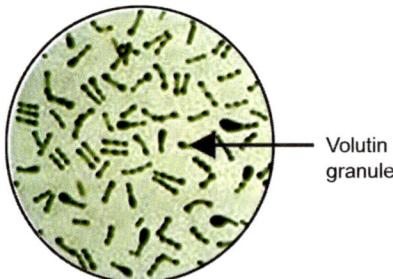

Fig. 14.1: *Corynebacterium diphtheriae* as seen after Albert staining

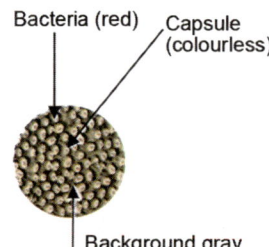

Fig. 15.4: *Visualization of capsule after staining the cell with safranin and background with India ink*

Plate 3

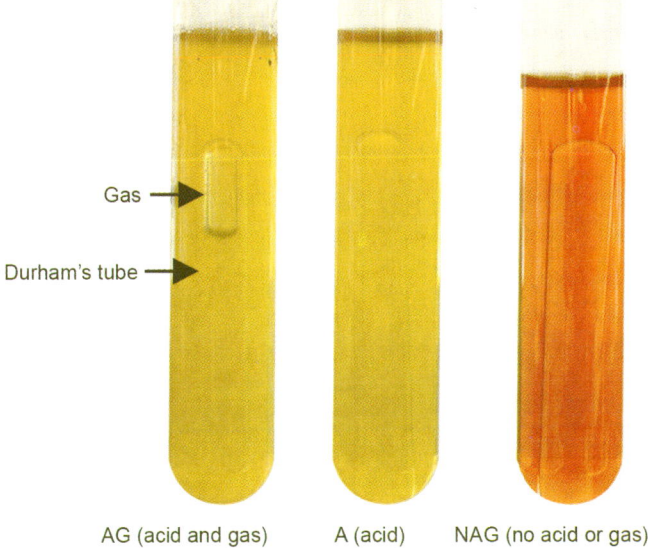

Fig. 19.12A: Carbohydrate fermentation test

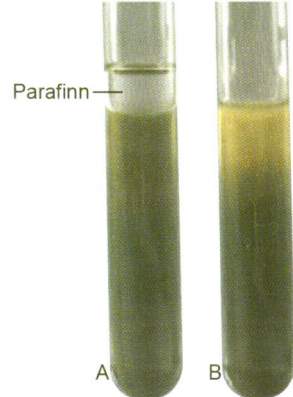

Oxidative utilization of carbohydrate in the open tube

Fig. 19.4: Carbohydrate oxidation-fermentation test: (A) No utilization of carbohydrate, (B) Oxidative utilization of carbohydrate

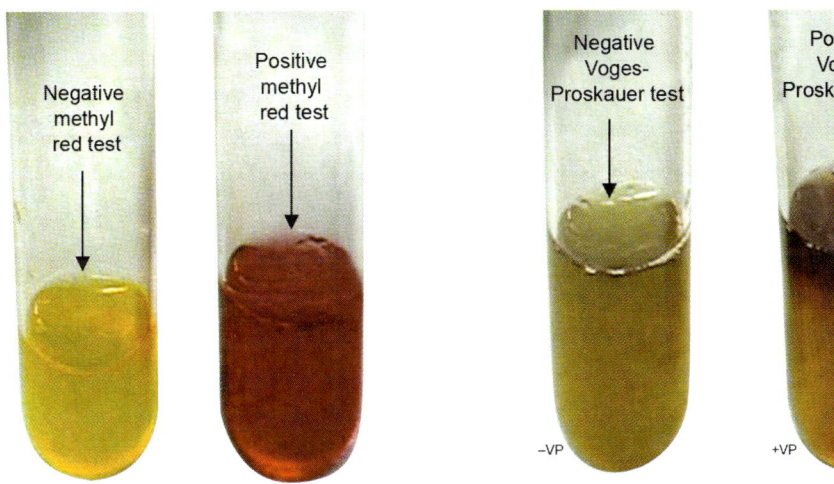

Fig. 19.5: Demonstration of methyl red test   **Fig. 19.7:** Demonstration of Voges-Proskauer test

Plate 4

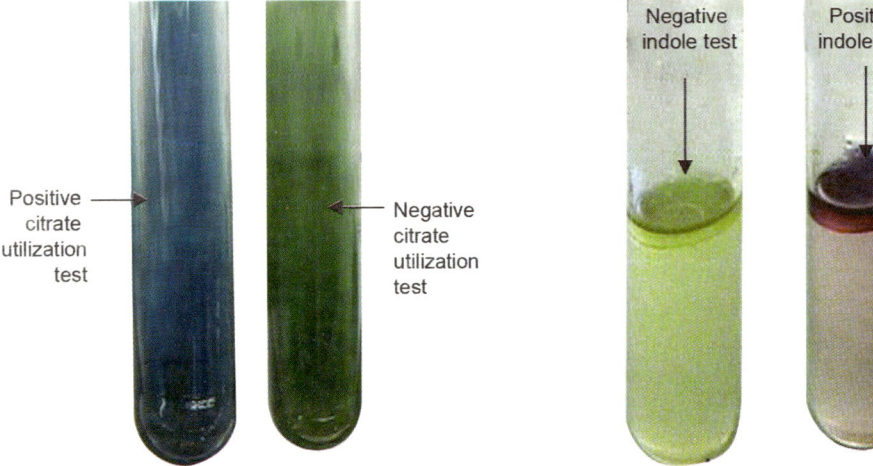

Fig. 19.9: Demonstration of citrate utilization test

Fig. 19.11: Demonstration of indole test

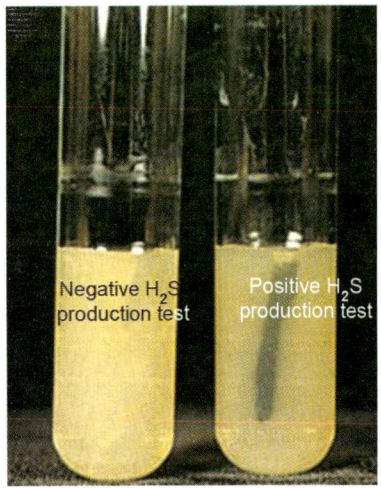

Fig. 19.13: Demonstration of H₂S production test

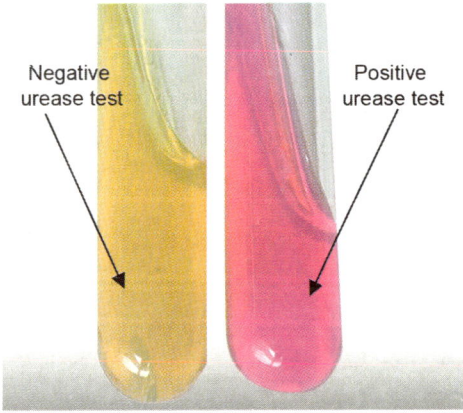

Fig. 19.14: Demonstration of urease production test

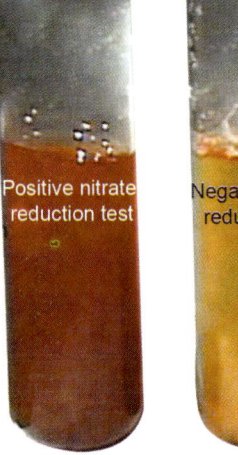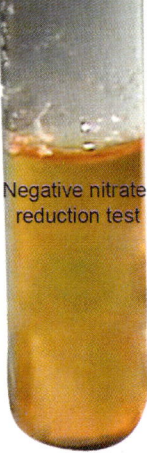

Fig. 19.16: Demonstration of nitrate reduction test

Plate 5

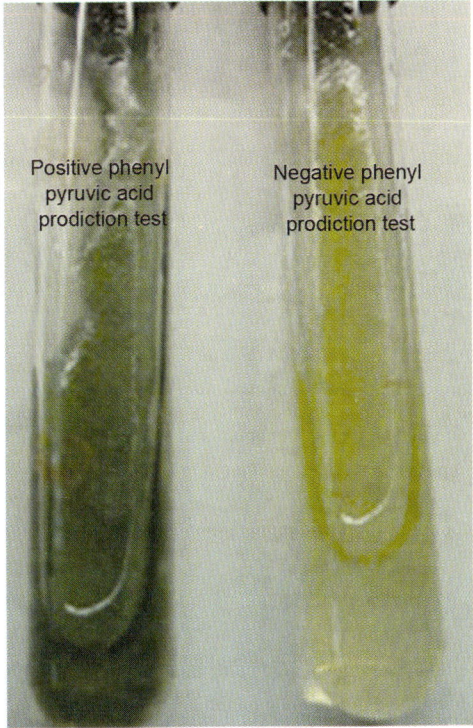

Fig. 19.18: Demonstration of positive and negative phenylpyruvic acid production test

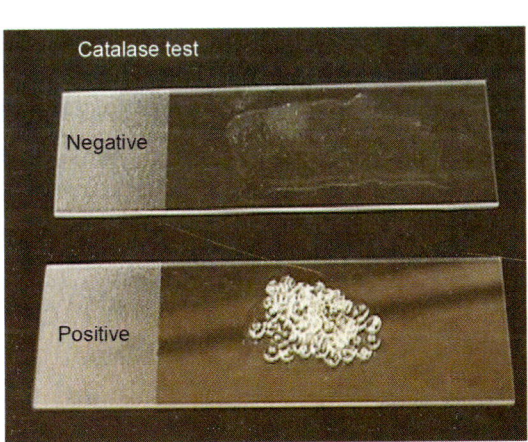

Fig. 19.20: Demonstration of catalase test

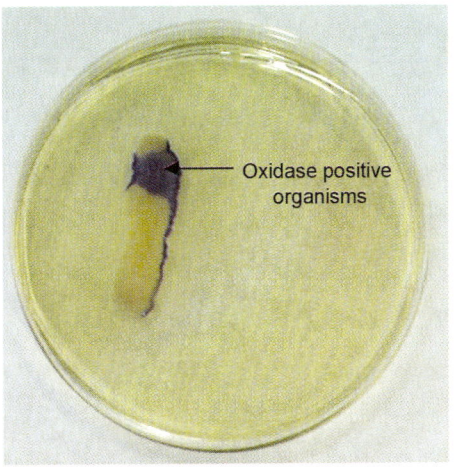

Fig. 19.22: Demonstration of oxidase test

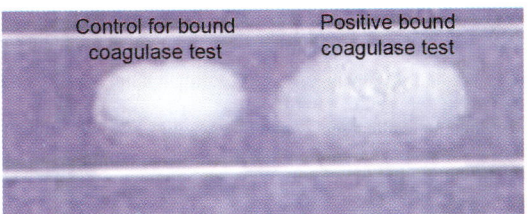

Fig. 19.23: Demonstration of bound coagulase test

Plate 6

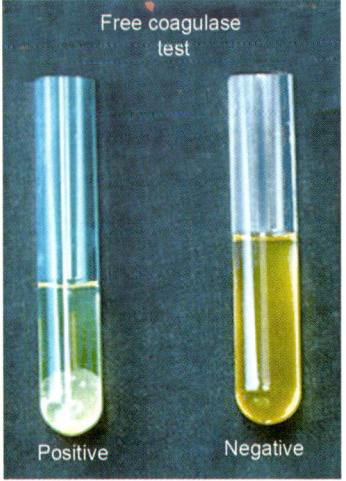

Fig. 19.24: Demonstration of free coagulase test

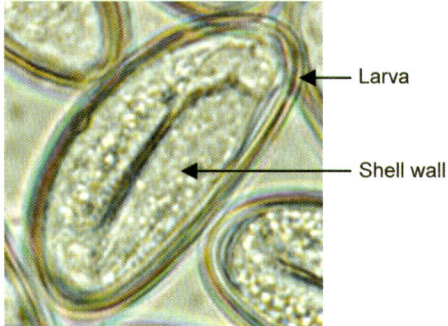

Fig. 32.4: (A) Pinworm (*Enterobius vermicularis*) ovum

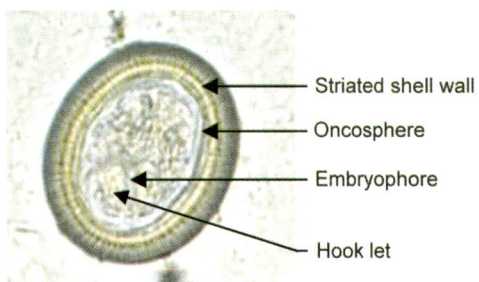

Fig. 32.4: (B) Tapeworm (*Taenia saginata/ Taenia solium*) ovum

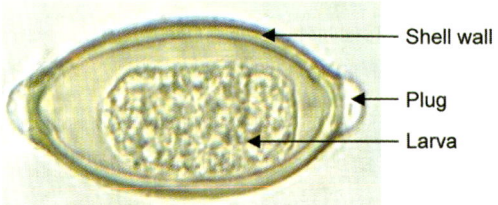

Fig. 32.4: (C) Whipworm (*Trichuris trichiura*) ovum

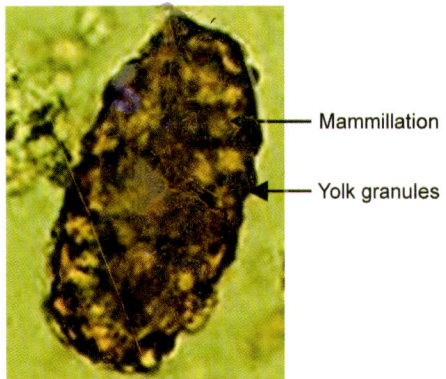

Fig. 32.4: (D) (i) Unfertilized roundworm (*Ascaris lumbricoides*) ovum

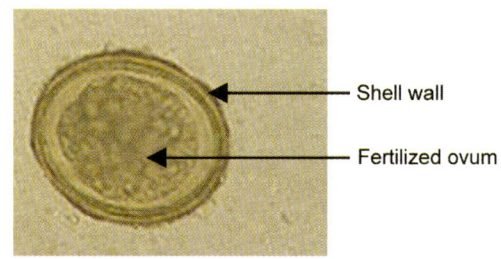

Fig. 32.4: (D) (ii) Decorticated and fertilized egg of roundworm

Plate 7

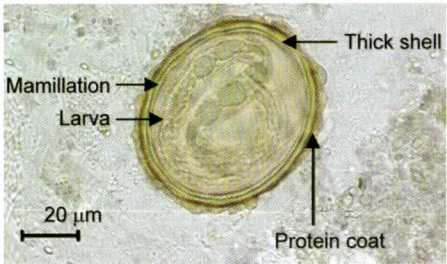

Fig. 32.4: (D) (iii) Embryonated roundworm ovum

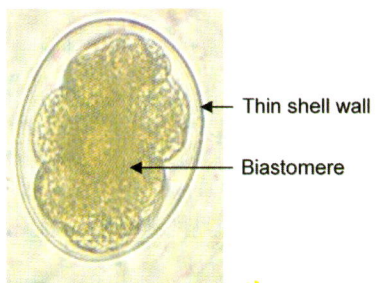

Fig. 32.4: (E) Hookworm (*Ancylostoma duodenale*) ovum

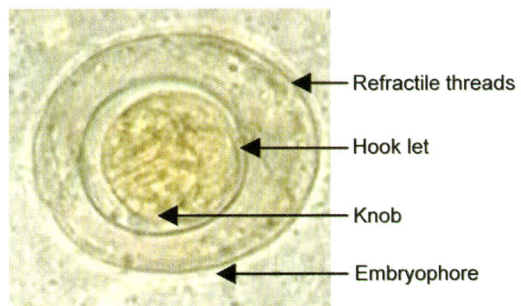

Fig. 32.4: (F) Dwarf tapeworm (*Hymenolepis nana*) ovum

Figs 32.4 (A to F): Identification of eggs of helminthes in fecal specimen

Observation

A positive test for nitrite production is indicated by development of red dye (Fig. 19.18).

Positive nitrate
reduction test

Negative nitrate
reduction test

Fig. 19.18: Demonstration of nitrate reduction test (*see* colour plate 4)

19.3.1.2 (e) Phenylpyruvic Acid Test or Phenylalanine Deaminase Test

Purpose

The phenylalanine deaminase test is used to differentiate the genera, *Proteus* and *Providencia* (phenylalanine deaminase-positive) from other members of the *Enterobacteriaceae* (phenylalanine deaminase-negative).

Principle

Phenylalanine deaminase tests demonstrate the ability of an organism to produce the enzyme phenaylalanine deaminase. This enzyme removes the amine group from the amino acid phenylalanine and releases it as free ammonia. As a result of this reaction, phenylpyruvic acid is also produced. Ferric chloride, when added to phenyl pyruvic acid, produces a dark green colour (Fig 19.19).

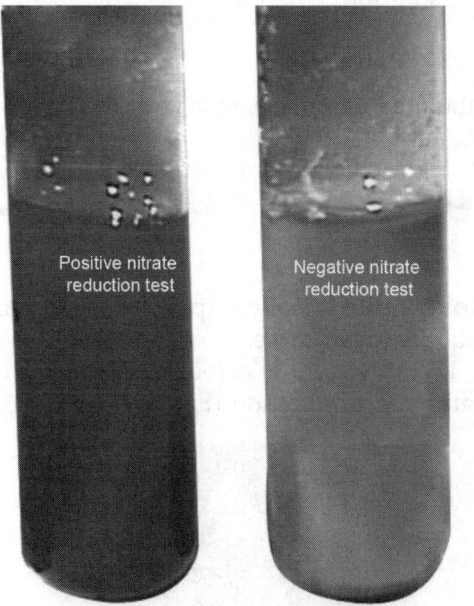

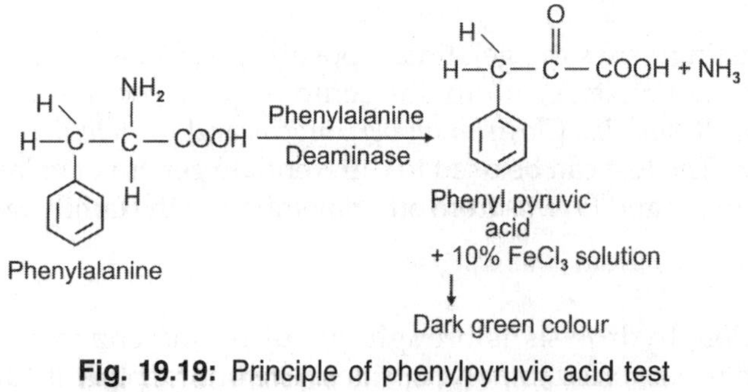

Fig. 19.19: Principle of phenylpyruvic acid test

Materials Required

- Sterile phenylalanine deaminase agar medium distributed in tubes as long slants.
- Pure culture of *Escherichia coli* and *Proteus vulgaris*.
- 10% ferric chloride solution.

Procedure

1. Inoculate phenylalanine deaminase agar with the bacteria.
2. Incubate overnight at 37°C.
3. Add 0.1 ml of 10% ferric chloride solution to the culture, mix well.
4. Examine the tubes.

Observation

- A dark green colour indicates phenylpyruvic acid production, i.e. organism produces phenylalanine deaminase.
- No colour change, i.e. straw yellow colour indicates the organism is negative for phenylalanine deaminase production (Fig. 19.20).

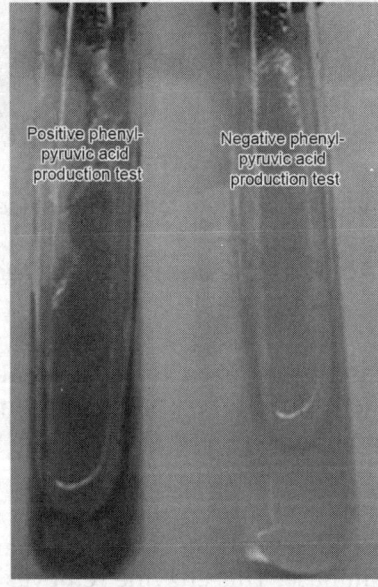

Positive phenyl-pyruvic acid production test

Negative phenyl-pyruvic acid production test

Fig. 19.20: Demonstration of positive and negative phenylpyruvic acid production test (*see* colour plate 5)

19.3.1.2 (f) Gelatin Liquefaction Test

Purpose

Gelatinase test distinguishes the gelatinase-positive, pathogenic *Staphylococcus aureus* from the gelatinase-negative, nonpathogenic *Staphylococcus epidermidis*. *Bacillus anthracis, B. cereus, B. subtilis, Clostridium perfringens* and *Cl. tetani* are also positive for gelatin hydrolysis. The test can be used to differentiate genera of gelatinase-producing bacteria such as *Serratia* and *Proteus* from other members of the family Enterobacteriaceae.

Principle

Gelatin liquefaction/hydrolysis is brought about by the enzyme gelatinase. In the first stage, gelatin is converted to polypeptides. The polypeptide is further hydrolysed to amino acids. Digested gelatin is no longer able to gel resulting in the liquefaction of the medium.

$$\text{Gelatin} \xrightarrow{\text{(Gelatinase)}} \text{Polypeptide} \longrightarrow \text{Amino acid}$$

Materials Required

- Sterile nutrient gelatin stab.
- Organism.

Preparation of nutrient gelatin

Ingredient	Preparation
• Peptone 5.0 g • Beef extract 3.0 g • Gelatin 120.0 g • Distilled water/deionized water 1 litre • Final pH: 6.8 ± 0.2 at 25°C.	1. Add the ingredients to 1,000 ml of distilled or deionized water and heat gently to dissolve. 2. Dispense 2 to 3 ml of medium into 13 mm × 100 mm culture tubes. 3. Autoclave medium at 121°C (15 psi) for 15 minutes. 4. Allow the tubed medium to cool in an upright position before use. 5. Store the prepared medium at 2 to 8°C.

Procedure

1. Stab inoculate the nutrient gelatin stabs with a heavy inoculum of desired organism(s). Keep some control tubes without inoculation.
2. Incubate the inoculated tubes and un-inoculated control tube at 25°C or at optimum growth temperature of the organism for up to one week.
3. Examine for liquefaction every day.
4. In case the tubes are incubated at a temperature of 28°C or higher, place the tubes in ice bath for 15 to 20 minutes
5. Examine for liquefaction.

Observation

In gelatinase-positive bacterium, the secreted gelatinases will hydrolyze the gelatin resulting in the liquefaction of the medium. Digested gelatin is no longer able to gel, the medium remains liquid when placed inside a refrigerator or in an ice bath. A

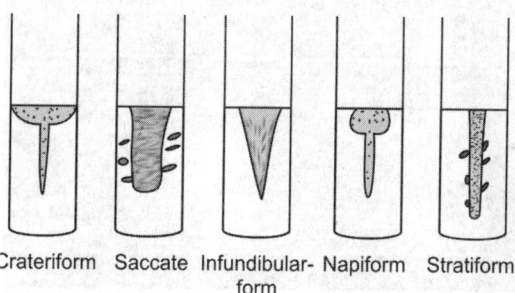

Crateriform   Saccate   Infundibular-   Napiform   Stratiform
form

Fig. 19.21: Forms of gelatin liquefaction

nutrient gelatin medium inoculated with a gelatinase-negative bacterium will remain solid after the cold treatment. Pattern of liquefaction helps in the identification of the organism (Fig. 19.21).

19.3.2 TESTS FOR SPECIFIC ENZYME PRODUCTION

19.3.2 (a) Catalase Test

Purpose: Catalase test is essential for differentiating catalase-positive *Micrococcaceae* from catalase-negative *Streptococcaceae*. Catalase test is also valuable in differentiating *Clostridium*, which are catalase negative, from *Bacillus*, which are catalase positive.

Principle

Catalase test demonstrate the ability of an organism to produce the enzyme catalase. This enzyme catalyses release of oxygen from hydrogen peroxide.

$$2H_2O_2 \xrightarrow{\text{(Catalase)}} 2H_2O + O_2$$

Materials Required

- Pure culture of *Streptococcus viridians* and *Staphylococcus* **on any medium except blood agar medium.**
- 3% hydrogen peroxide.

Procedure

1. Pour 1 ml of hydrogen peroxide over a 24 hours nutrient agar slope cultures of the organisms.
2. Examine for gas production in the tube.

Observation

- Production of gas bubbles indicates that organisms are positive for catalase test, i.e. they can produce catalase.
- No gas bubbles indicates that organisms are negative for catalase test, i.e. they cannot produce catalase (Fig. 19.22).

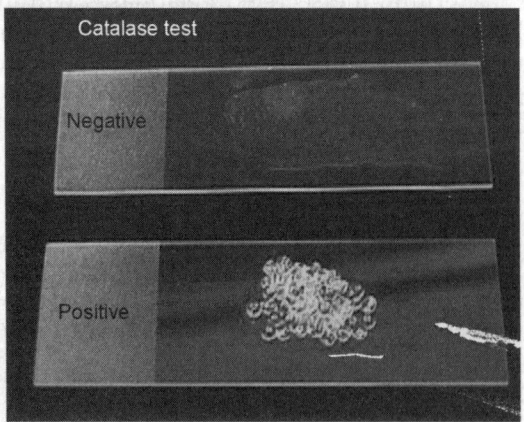

Fig. 19.22: Demonstration of catalase test (*see* colour plate 5)

19.3.2. (b) Oxidase Test

Purpose

Oxidase test is done to distinguish *Neisseria gonorrhoeae* (oxidase positive) from *Staphylococcus* spp and *Streptococcus* spp (oxidase negative) and also to differentiate *Pseudomonas* spp from other Gram-negative rods.

Principle

Oxidase (cytochrome oxidase) test demonstrates the ability of an organism to produce the enzyme cytochrome oxidase, which catalyzes the oxidation of cytochrome *c* (one of the components in the electron transport chain of bacteria) (Fig. 19.23). For carrying out the oxidase test, tetra-methyl-*p*-phenylene diamine dihydrochloride, is used as an artificial electron donor for cytochrome *c*. When this colourless reagent is oxidized by cytochrome *c oxidase*, it changes its colour to dark blue or purple due to its oxidized state of indophenol blue.

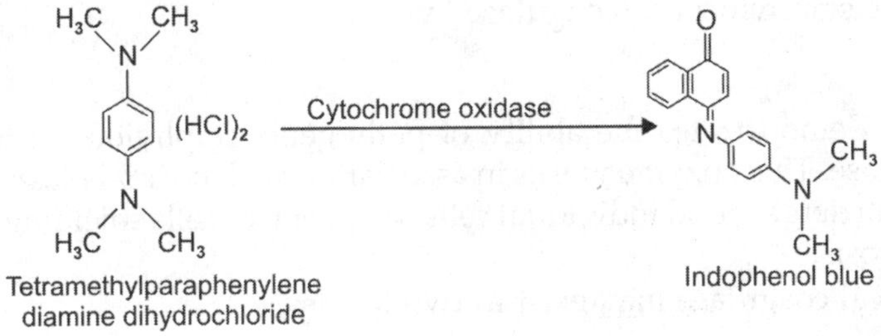

Tetramethylparaphenylene diamine dihydrochloride → Cytochrome oxidase → Indophenol blue

Fig. 19.23: Principle of oxidase test

Materials Required
- Pure culture of *Escherichia coli* and *Pseudomonas aeruginosa* on any medium.
- Freshly prepared 1% solution of tetramethylparaphenylene diamine dihydrochloride in distilled water.
- Inoculating loop made of an inert material (**no iron loop**).

Procedure
1. Soak a filter paper strip with the freshly prepared reagent.
2. Rub a speck of culture on the filter paper strip with the loop of an inert (platinum) material.
3. Observe the rubbed material within 10 seconds.

Observation
- Production of deep purple colour (colour of oxidized state of the reagent) indicates that organisms are positive for oxidase test, i.e. they can produce oxidase enzyme.
- No colour production within 10 seconds indicates that organisms are negative for oxidase test, i.e. they cannot produce oxidase enzyme (Fig. 19.24).

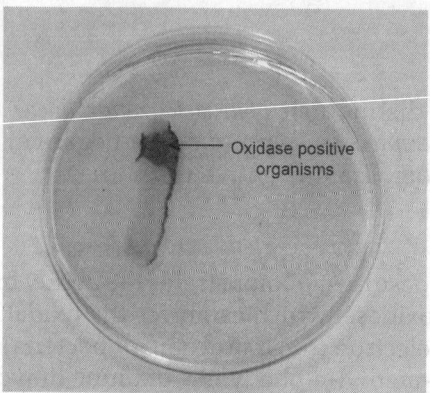

Fig. 19.24: Demonstration of oxidase test (*see* colour plate 5)

19.3.2 (c) Coagulase Test

Purpose

Coagulase test is done to differentiate pathogenic staphylococci (coagulase +ve) from non-pathogenic staphylococci (coagulase –ve).

Principle

Coagulase test demonstrates the ability of pathogenic staphylococci to produce the enzyme coagulase. This enzyme works in association with normal plasma components to form fibrin barriers around individual cells or a group of cells shielding the organisms from phagocytosis.

Staphylococcal coagulase may exist in two forms.

1. Bound coagulase (also called clumping factor) that is attached to the bacterial cell wall and reacts directly with the plasma fibrinogen to form clumps of cells trapped within fibrin threads.
2. Free coagulase that is an extracellular enzyme which activates and combines with a plasma coagulase-reacting factor (CRF)—a modified or derived thrombin molecule. This coagulase–CRF complex, in turn, catalyzes the conversion of soluble fibrinogen to fibrin clots.

19.3.2 (c-i) Bound Coagulase Test

Materials Required

- Pure culture *Staphylococcus aureus* and *Staphylococcus epidermidis* on any medium.
- Human or rabbit plasma obtained from citrated or oxalated blood.
- Sterile 0.85% sodium chloride solution (physiological saline).

Procedure

1. Take a clean, grease free 3″ × 1 glass slide.
2. Mark into two parts with a marker.
3. Place a loopful of saline on each section and emulsify with the bacterial growth to get a homogeneous suspension of the bacteria in saline.
4. Add 1 drop of plasma on one part. The other part serves as a control.
5. Examine the slide for clumping of the suspension.

Observation

- Clumping only on the side where plasma has been added indicates that organisms are positive for coagulase test, i.e. they can produce coagulase enzyme (Fig. 19.25).

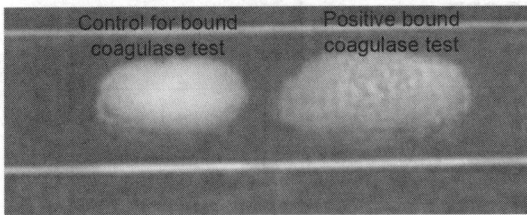

Fig. 19.25: Demonstration of bound coagulase test (*see* colour plate 5)

19.3.2 (c-ii) Free Coagulase Test

Materials Required

- 1:10 dilution of plasma.
- Broth cultures of known coagulase positive and coagulase negative bacterial strains.
- Broth culture of the test organism.

Procedure

1. Take three tubes. Mark them 1, 2 and 3.
2. Add 0.5 ml of diluted plasma in all three tubes.
3. To tube 1, add 0.5 ml of broth culture of coagulase negative organism.
4. To tube 2, add 0.5 ml of broth culture of coagulase positive organism.
5. To tube 3, add 0.5 ml of the test organism.
6. Incubate all tubes at 37°C.
7. Examine for clotting after 1 hour and at 30 minutes intervals up to 6 hours.

Observation

- There will be no clotting in tube no1.
- There will be clotting in tube no 2.
- Clotting in tube no 3 shall indicate that the test organism is coagulase positive. Absence of clotting in tube no 3 indicates that the organisms are coagulase negative (Fig. 19.26)

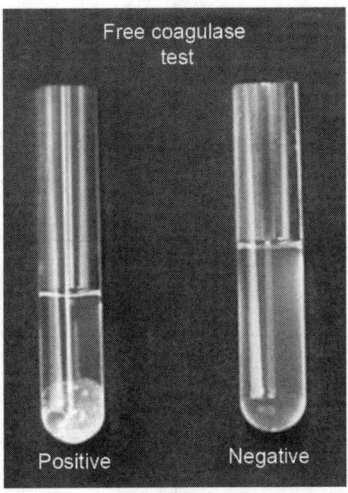

Fig. 19.26: Demonstration of free coagulase test (*see* colour plate 6)

19.4 LABORATORY RECORD

Perform biochemical tests on different organisms and record your observations.

Date	Name of the organism	Name of the biochemical test performed	Observation	Report	Teacher's signature

Testing Antimicrobial
Susceptibility of Bacteria: Kirby-Bauer Method

20.1 AIM

To educate the students about the importance of performing antimicrobial sensitivity test with each pathological isolate from the specimens and the method of conducting the test.

20.2 LEARNING OUTCOME

After this exercise, students are able to understand the purpose of doing antimicrobial sensitivity tests, different types of antimicrobial sensitivity tests used in the laboratories and can perform the tests at their level.

20.3 PURPOSE

Antimicrobial sensitivity test is conducted to detect possible drug resistance amongst common pathogens and to choose the appropriate drug for treating the particular infection.

20.4 METHODS

Methods used for performing antimicrobial susceptibility test include:
- Manual methods
- Automated methods

The manual methods of performing antimicrobial sensitivity tests are:
- Broth dilution method.
- Diffusion method.

Broth dilution method is mostly used for determining the **minimum inhibitory concentration (MIC)** of an antibiotic.

Automated methods are faster and more expensive. Available automated instruments namely, MicroScan WalkAway, BD Phoenix automated microbiology system, Vitek 2 system, etc. can simultaneously process 64 to 240 tests. Manufacturer's instructions are to be followed strictly while using these machines.

20.4.1 Principle of Agar Diffusion Method

When an antibiotic disc is placed on an agar surface pre-coated with the bacteria, simultaneous growth of the bacteria and diffusion of the antimicrobial compounds takes place. Concentration of the antibiotics reduces as the antibiotic diffuses away from the disc. In case the bacteria are killed by the antibiotic, a zone of inhibition is seen. The size of the zone of inhibition of growth is influenced by the depth of the agar and the number of organisms in the inoculum. Based on the diameter of zone of inhibition as compared with standard for each antibiotic used, qualitative information as susceptible, intermediate or resistant are given.

Different disc diffusion methods include the following:

20.4.1.1 Kirby-Bauer Method

In this method, the pathogenic organism is grown on Müller-Hinton agar in the presence of filter paper disks impregnated with various antimicrobial compounds. Absence of growth around the disks is an indirect measure of the ability of the antimicrobial compound to inhibit that organism (Fig. 20.1).

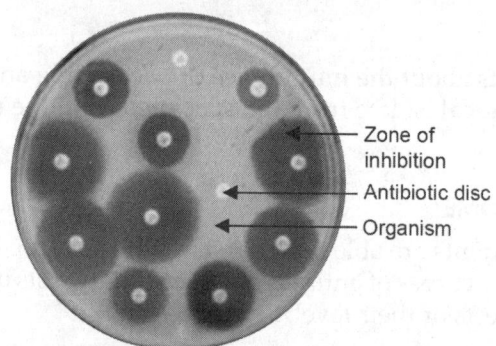

Fig. 20.1: Sensitivity plate (Kirby-Bauer method)

20.4.1.2 Stoke's Method

This method uses in-built control against many variables. In this method, the agar surface on the petridish is divided into three parts. The test organism is inoculated at the central part and the control organisms on the top and bottom parts. Antibiotic discs are placed on the lines separating the test organism. Comparison of results with the control organism is obtained in the same plate (Fig. 20.2).

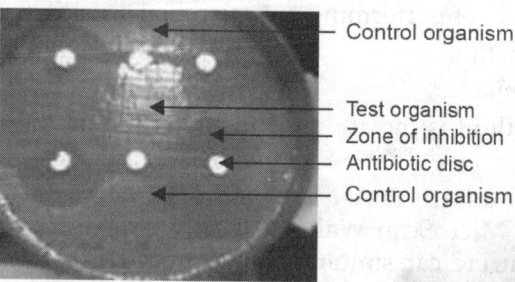

Fig. 20.2: Sensitivity plate (Stoke's method)

20.4.1.3 Epsilometer Test (E-Test)

This method uses a plastic disc having a continuous gradient of antibiotic coated on one side and the minimum inhibitory concentration (MIC) interpretative scale on other side. The disc is placed on the petridish pre-inoculated with the desired organism. MIC scale faces the opening side. After incubation, the antibiotic susceptibility along with the MIC can be seen (Fig. 20.3).

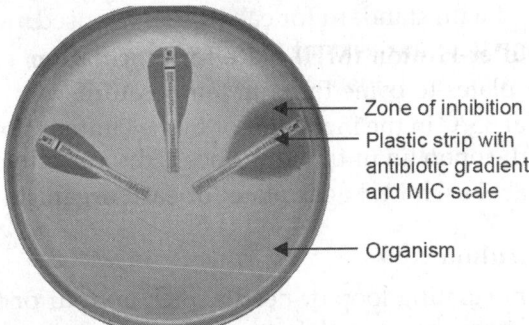

Zone of inhibition

Plastic strip with
antibiotic gradient
and MIC scale

Organism

Fig. 20.3: Sensitivity plate (E-test strip method)

20.5 PROCEDURE FOR KIRBY-BAUER METHOD

Kirby-Bauer method: The disk diffusion method of Kirby and Bauer has been standardized and is a viable method in the laboratories those do not have resources to utilize the automated methods.

20.5.1 Materials Required for Kirby-Bauer Method

- Antibiotic disks.
- Alcohol pads or isopropyl alcohol in a tube.
- Bunsen burner.
- Caliper or ruler.
- Forceps.
- 35°C to 37°C non-CO$_2$ incubator.
- Inoculating loop or needle.
- 0.5 McFarland standard.
- Sterile Müller-Hinton agar plates, (100 mm or 150 mm diameter).
- 18 to 24 hours old pure culture of the organism to be tested.
- Sterile saline in 2 ml tubes.
- Sterile swabs.
- Vortex mixer.

Antibiotic disks: Antimicrobial disks can be purchased from any reputed suppliers.

Preparation of McFarland Standard

A 0.5 McFarland standard is equivalent to a bacterial suspension containing between 1×10^8 and 2×10^8 colony forming unit (CFU)/ml of *Escherichia coli*. It can be prepared in house as follows:

1. Add a 0.5 ml aliquot of a 0.048 mol/liter BaCl$_2$ (1.175% wt/volume BaCl$_2$-2H$_2$0) to 99.5 ml of 0.18 mol/liter H$_2$SO$_4$ (1% vol/vol) with constant stirring to maintain a suspension.
2. Verify the correct density of the turbidity standard by measuring absorbance using a spectrophotometer with a 1 cm light path and a matched cuvette. The absorbance at 625 nm should be between 0.08 and 0.13 for the 0.5 McFarland standard.
3. Transfer the barium sulfate suspension in 4 to 6 ml aliquots into screw-cap tubes of the same size as those used for standardizing the bacterial inoculum.
4. Tightly seal the tubes and store in the dark at room temperature.
5. Prior to use, vigorously agitate the barium sulfate standard on a mechanical vortex mixer and inspect for a uniformly turbid appearance. Discard the standard if large particles appear.

Procedure

A. Preparation of Müller-Hinton (MH) plate for inoculation

1. Allow MH agar plates to come to room temperature.
2. Place the plates at 35°C in the incubator or in the laminar flow hood inverting the agar surface on the open lid until the surface is dry (usually for 10 to 30 minutes).
3. Appropriately label each MH agar plate for each organism to be tested.

B. Preparation of inoculum

1. Using a sterile inoculating loop or needle, pick up four or five isolated colonies of the organism from the agar plate.
2. Suspend the organism in 2 ml of sterile saline.
3. Vortex the saline tube to create a smooth suspension.
4. Adjust the turbidity of this suspension to a 0.5 McFarland standard by adding more organism if the suspension is too light or diluting with sterile saline if the suspension is too heavy.
5. Use this suspension within 15 minutes of preparation.

C. Inoculation of the MH plate

1. Dip a sterile swab into the inoculum tube.
2. Remove excess fluid from the swab by rotating the swab against the side of the tube (above the fluid level) using firm pressure.
3. Inoculate the dried surface of the MH agar plate by streaking the swab three times over the entire agar surface ensuring an even distribution of the inoculum.
4. Pick up any excessive inoculums that may have splashed near the edge by running the swab around the edge of the entire the plate.
5. Discard the swab into an appropriate container with disinfectant.
6. Leave the lid slightly open and allow the plate to sit at room temperature at least for 3 to 5 minutes, but no more than 15 minutes, in order to dry the surface of the agar plate.

D. Placement of the antibiotic disks

1. Place the appropriate antimicrobial-impregnated disks on the surface of the agar, using sterile forceps. Sterilize the forceps by cleaning them with a sterile alcohol pad and allowing them to air dry or immersing the forceps in alcohol then flaming.
2. Carefully remove one disk from the cartridge using the forceps.
3. Partially open the lid of the petridish. Place the disk on the plate and gently press the disk with the forceps to ensure complete contact with the agar surface. Close the petridish lid to minimize exposure of the agar surface to room air.
4. Continue to place one disk at a time onto the agar surface until all disks have been placed.
5. Once all disks are in place, replace the lid, invert the plates, and place them in an incubator at 35°C for 16 to 18 hours.

E. Measuring zone sizes (Fig. 20.4)

1. After the incubation, take out the petridish, and, viewing the back side of the plate, measure the zone sizes with unaided eyes using a ruler or caliper. Hold the plate a few inches above a black, nonreflecting surface illuminated with reflected light. Include the diameter of the disk in the measurement (Fig. 20.4).

2. When measuring zone diameters, always round up to the next millimeter avoiding any parallax by holding the plate using a direct, vertical line of sight.
3. Record the zone size on the recording sheet.
4. Report growth up to the edge of the disk as a zone of 0 mm.
5. For organisms such as *Proteus mirabilis*, which swarm, ignore the thin veil of swarming and measure the outer margin in an otherwise obvious zone of inhibition.

Interpretation and reporting of the antibiotic susceptibility results
1. Using the published Clinical and Laboratory Standard Institute (CLSI) guidelines, determine the susceptibility or resistance of the organism to each drug tested.
2. Based on the interpretation chart for each drug, indicate on the recording sheet whether the zone size is susceptible (S), intermediate (I), or resistant (R).
3. The results of the Kirby-Bauer disk diffusion susceptibility test are reported only as susceptible, intermediate, or resistant. Zone sizes are not reported to physicians.

20.6 QUALITY CONTROL

- Recommended organisms for quality assurance purposes are *Staphylococcus aureus* ATCC 25923, *Escherichia coli* ATCC 25922 and *Pseudomonas aeruginosa* ATCC 27853, as the zone of inhibition for these organisms is known (ATCC: American Type Culture Collection)

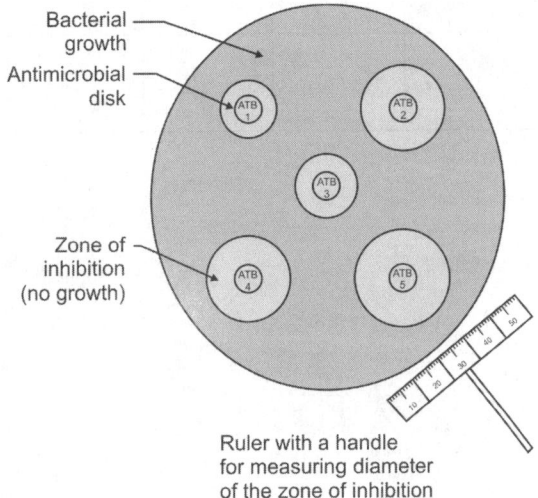

Fig. 20.4: Measurement of zone of inhibition

- Select the antimicrobial compound based on the type of organism being tested and source of the isolate (blood, urine, wound, etc.).
- Test the MH agar medium with known strains of organism every week in order to verify that the media and disks are working as expected.
- For testing the organism, take the inoculum when the organisms are in the log phase of growth.
- While reading the plates, ensure that there is a confluent lawn of growth and the zones of inhibition are uniformly circular.
- Consider the zone margin as the area showing no visible growth that can be detected with the unaided eye. Do not use a magnification device to observe zone edges.

20.7 LABORATORY RECORDS

Perform antimicrobial susceptibility tests with pure culture of organisms and record your observation

Date	Organism	Antimicrobial sensitivity test report					Teacher's signature
		Name of antibiotic 1	Name of antibiotic 2	Name of antibiotic 3	Name of antibiotic 4	Name of antibiotic 5	

Isolation and Identification of Pure Bacterial Cultures

21.1 AIM

To teach the students the methods used for isolation of common organisms in pure culture and their subsequent identification by examining their colony characteristics, Gram staining, motility and biochemical reactions.

21.2 LEARNING OUTCOME

The students learns various methods used for isolating organisms in pure culture, are able to isolate organisms in a pure culture by streak plate method and can identify the organisms by examining their colony characteristics, Gram staining, motility and biochemical reactions.

21.3 METHODS FOR ISOLATION OF PURE BACTERIAL CULTURES

Methods for isolating bacteria in a pure culture from a mixed one includes the following:
- **Surface plating** by the use of streak plate method.
- **Filtration** by using filters according to the size of the cells.
- **Using enrichment and selective medium.**
- **Separation of motile and non-motile bacteria** by using tools like Craigies tube.
- **Using selective growth conditions,** e.g. temperature, pH, oxygen concentration, salt concentration, etc.
- **Animal inoculation** (not done except for research purpose).

Out of above methods, **streak plate method** is used routinely for picking up an isolated colony and subsequently growing it in broth for its rapid growth.

21.4 IDENTIFICATION OF ORGANISMS

Preliminary identification of the organisms is based on:
- Macroscopic examination of growth and colony characteristics in the medium.
- Microscopic examination for Gram staining and motility.
- Biochemical reactions.

Subsequent confirmation may include
- Examination on the basis of toxin production.
- Immunological methods of identification.

21.5 ISOLATION OF ORGANISMS BY STREAK PLATE METHOD AND THEIR FURTHER IDENTIFICATION

21.5.1 Materials Required

- One nutrient agar, one MacConkey agar plate and one blood agar plate.
- Inoculating loop.

- Overnight growth of the organisms in a mixed culture.
- Incubator.
- Microscope.
- Gram staining reagents.
- Various media for conducting biochemical tests.
- Slides and cover slips.

21.5.2 Procedure

1. Take the overnight broth culture of different organisms with sterile inoculating loop.
2. Inoculate aseptically on one nutrient agar one MacConkey agar and one blood agar plate.
3. Incubate overnight at 37°C.
4. Examine the isolated colonies appearing on the agar plate for their general growth character and individual colony characteristics.
5. Take a single colony and inoculate into a peptone water media.
6. Touch one of the well isolated colonies with a sterile inoculating loop and do the Gram staining with the picked up growth.
7. Incubate for two hours.
8. Transfer one loopful from the peptone water culture of the organism to each of the medium used for doing biochemical tests for examining their utilization of carbohydrate and nitrogen containing materials.
9. Incubate overnight.
10. Examine the results of their biochemical activities on the next day.

21.5.3 Observation with Known Organisms

Gram character and morphology	Motility	Major growth character	Major colony characteristics	Biochemical reactions	Name of the organism
Gram-negative rods	Sluggishly motile	Lactose fermenting on MacConkey agar	Rose pink colonies	Indole +ve. Methyl red +ve. Carbohydrate fermentation – AG production. H₂S production +ve. VP –ve. Citrate utilization –ve.	Escherichia coli
Gram-negative rods	Non-motile	Lactose fermenting on MacConkey agar	Pink, mucoid colonies	Indole –ve. Methyl red –ve. Carbohydrate fermentation AG production. H₂S production – ve. VP+ve. Citrate utilization +ve. Urease +ve.	Klebsiella
Gram-negative rods	Actively motile	Non-lactose fermenting on	Flat colonies	Oxidase positive.	Pseudomonas

(Contd.)

(Contd.)

Gram character and morphology	Motility	Major growth character	Major colony characteristics	Biochemical reactions	Name of the organism
		MacConkey agar, soluble green pigment with aromatic odour in all media			
Gram-negative rods	Actively motile	Non-lactose fermenting colonies on MacConkey agar	Swarming growth on BA medium and NA media	Urease positive. PPA + ve.	*Proteus*
Gram-positive cocci in clusters	Non-motile	Light yellow to yellow coloured colony on NA, complete hemolysis on BA medium Non-lactose fermenting on MacConkey agar	Smooth, opaque colonies with convex elevation, insoluble pigment	Mannitol fermentation +ve. Urease +ve. Catalase +ve. Coagulase +ve.	*Staphylococcus aureus*
Gram-positive cocci in clusters	Non-motile	White colony on NA, complete hemolysis on BA medium. Non-lactose fermenting on MacConkey agar	Smooth, opaque colonies with convex elevation, insoluble pigment	Urease +ve. Catalase +ve. Coagulase –ve.	*Staphylococcus albus*
Gram-positive cocci in chains	Non-motile	Very small colonies with greenish zone of incomplete hemolysis on BA medium	Smooth, very small colonies	Catalase –ve	*Streptococcus viridans*
Gram-positive cocci in chains	Non-motile	Very small colonies with clear zone of complete hemolysis on BA medium	Smooth, very small colonies	Catalase –ve	*Streptococcus pyogenes*

21.6 LABORATORY RECORD

1. Take different specimens.
2. Isolate the organisms in pure culture.
3. Perform Gram staining and put up biochemical tests.
4. Record results of Gram staining, cultural characteristics and biochemical reactions as follows:

Date	Sample	Morphology, gram reaction and motility	Growth and colony characteristics	Results of biochemical reaction	Organism identified	Teacher's signature

General Guidelines for Collection and Transport of Clinical Specimens for Bacteriological Examination

22.1 AIM

To create awareness amongst students on general guidelines on proper collection for of clinical specimens and their transportation to the laboratory so as to achieve a reliable diagnosis.

22.2 LEARNING OUTCOME

The students understand the importance of having a properly collected, identified and transported clinical specimen in the laboratory for diagnosis of an infectious disease.

22.3 PURPOSE OF CONDUCTING BACTERIOLOGICAL DIAGNOSIS OF A CLINICAL SPECIMEN

- To find out the organism responsible for the disease.
- To find out the best antibiotics for treatment of the disease.
- To assess whether the treatment has been fruitful or not.

22.4 STEPS FOR PROCESSING A CLINICAL SPECIMEN FOR BACTERIOLOGICAL DIAGNOSIS

- Collection of right clinical specimen at right time.
- Proper transportation of the specimen with proper identification(labeling).
- Acceptance of the specimen in the laboratory.
- Macroscopic examination of the specimen.
- Microscopic examination.
- Cultivation and isolation in pure culture.
- Identification of the causative organism by various methods.
- Antimicrobial susceptibility testing.

22.4.1 Collection of Clinical Specimen

WHO recommended general rules for collection of a clinical specimen are as follows:
- Collect the specimen before administration of any antimicrobial agent.
- Follow strict aseptic procedure to prevent contamination of the specimen with externally present organisms or normal flora of the body.
- Wash hands before and after collecting the specimen.
- Ensure that the specimen is a proper representative of the infectious process.
- Collect the specimen at the appropriate phase of the disease.
- Collect/place the specimen aseptically in a sterile/appropriate container.
- Ensure that outside of the specimen container is clean and not soiled.

- Close the container tightly so that the contents do not leak during transportation.
- Label and date the container appropriately and complete the requisition form.
- Arrange for immediate transportation to the laboratory.

22.4.2 Transportation of the Specimen to the Laboratory (Fig. 22.1)

Pack the specimen safely. In some cases, e.g. in case of stool sample, use transport medium.

For hand—carried transportation over a short distance, place the specimen upright in appropriate racks.

For long distance transportation, use following three containers:

1. A leak proof primary container with a screw cap in which the specimen is placed.
2. A durable, waterproof secondary metal or a plastic container with a screw cap having enough absorptive material to absorb the content of the primary container in case leakage or breakage of the primary container occurs. Paste the details of the specimen on the outside of the secondary container.
3. A tertiary container made of wood or cardboard capable of withstanding the shock of transportation.

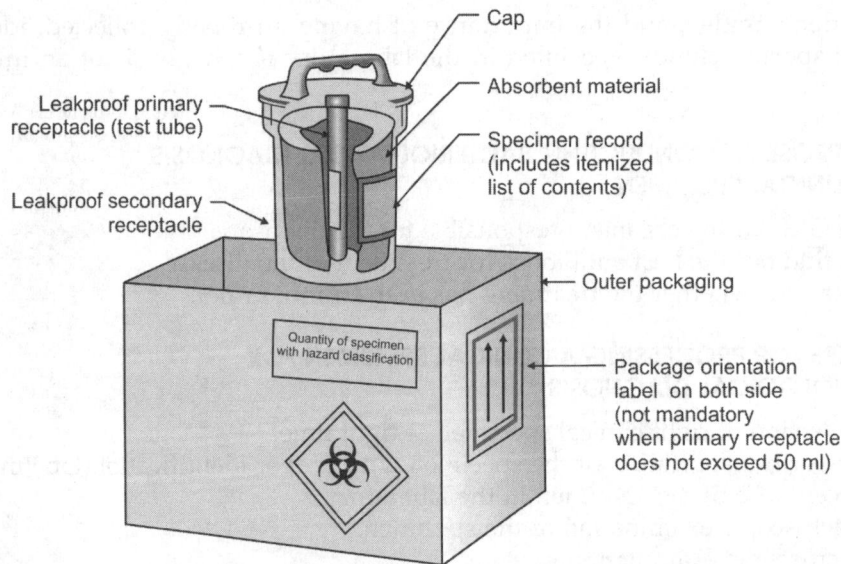

Fig. 22.1: Packaging for transportation of specimen according to CDC guideline

22.4.3 Acceptance of the Specimen

Accept the specimen for processing in the laboratory after ensuring the following:

- Proper labeling of the specimen.
- Sufficient quantity of the specimen.
- Specimen collected in appropriate container.
- Appropriate transport and storage of the specimen
- Collection time indicated.
- No contamination suspected.
- Blood sample without hemolysis.

In general, most specimens should be processed in the laboratory within 1–2 hours after collection.

22.5 LABORATORY RECORD

Check the container of the specimen received in your laboratory. Record your observation as under:

Date	Type of specimen received	Precautions taken during collection/receipt of specimen	Whether accepted for culture or not	Reason for rejection, if any	Teacher's signature

23

Route from Patient to Microbial Diagnosis

23.1 AIM

To give an overview to the students on the steps to be followed while processing specimens for bacteriological diagnosis.

23.2 LEARNING OUTCOME

Students become aware of the step by step procedures to be followed for processing the specimens for bacteriological diagnosis of an infectious disease.

For laboratories with automation, follow the manufacturer's instructions carefully while processing the sample.

General steps followed in processing the specimens for microbiological diagnosis are given in Table 23.1 as under:

Table 23.1: General steps for processing the specimens

Day	Activity	Remarks
Day 1	Collect sample.Label the sample. Send to the laboratory following the guidelines on transportation.	Procedure may be done in the patient care unit or in the laboratory
Day 1	Receive the sample in the laboratory. Accept the specimen after checking the label on the container, quality of the container and the specimen quality. Do macroscopic evaluation of the specimen based on odour, consistency, etc. Do microscopic examination of the specimen taking every precaution against possible contamination of the specimen. Put up culture for isolation of the organism. Select appropriate growth medium, temperature and environment for incubation. Put up supplementary tests like capsule swelling, antigen antibody reactions, DNA detection by PCR (if facilities are available), etc.	Give preliminary report to the physician based on macroscopic examination and microscopic examination
Day 2 or subsequent days	Isolate the organism in pure culture. Identify the organism by biochemical tests. Interpret whether organisms are contaminants, commensal or pathogens.	Give final report to the physician.
	Put up antimicrobial sensitivity test.	
Day 3 and subsequent days	Check the antimicrobial sensitivity report.	Send antibiotic sensitivity report to the physician.

Processing of Urine Samples for Culture and Antibiotic Sensitivity

24.1 AIM

To educate the students the importance of urine as a specimen for the diagnosis of urinary tract infection and the correct procedure for its collection, culture and sensitivity so as to reach a confirmatory diagnosis.

24.2 LEARNING OUTCOME

Students learn to advise the patients on correct procedure for urine collection and can perform the urine culture and sensitivity test efficiently.

24.3 PURPOSE

Urine is the specimen for diagnosis of urinary tract infection (UTI), i.e. infection in any part of the urinary tract namely, kidney, ureter, bladder and urethra (Fig. 24.1).

Under normal condition, bladder, ureter and kidney are sterile. The lower part of the urethra and genitalia are normally colonized by bacteria some of which may also cause UTI.

24.4 PATHOGENS AND CONTAMINANTS

Pathogen	Contaminant (from urethra and surrounding skin)
Most common agents for UTI are *Escherichia coli, Klbsiella,* other organisms include *Proteus, Pseudomonas, Streptococcus faecalis, citrobacter.* Less common isolates are *Staphylococcus aureus,* beta hemolytic streptococci, *Mycobacterium, Salmonella, Candida,* etc.	Diphtheroids, intestinal organisms in small number, coagulase negative staphylococci, etc.

24.5 COLLECTION

For microbiological examination, morning urine sample is preferred. For collection of a clean catch, mid-stream urine (to avoid contamination with surface colonizing bacteria and epithelial cells) sample, following steps are taken:

For adult men and women: Patients must first wash their hands thoroughly and then wash the penis or vulva and surrounding area four times, with front-to-back strokes, using a new soapy sponge each time.

The patient must then begin urinating into the toilet for a while.
- The patient then positions the sterile container to catch the middle portion of the stream without touching any part of the body and collect the urine in the container without soiling the outside of the container.

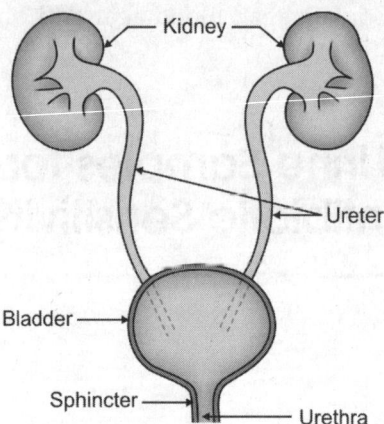

Fig. 24.1: Urinary tract

- The patient securely screws the container cap in place without touching the inside of the rim.

For Infants

- Wash the infant's genitalia with sponge soaked in mild soap solution. Repeat three times.
- Place the infant in a face down position and collect the mid-stream urine. Alternatively, place a sterile bag over the genitalia of the infant and collect a spontaneous sample.

The specimen must reach the laboratory within one hour of collection. In case of delay, place it in the refrigerator at 4°C.

24.6 EXAMINATION OF THE URINE SAMPLE

24.6.1 Automated System

- MS 2 system uses cuvettes and principle of nephelometry for urine culture.
- Automicrobic system uses tiny wells for urine culture.
- Bac-T-screens uses filter papers for detection of bacteriuria.

In all cases, manufacturer's instructions are to be followed carefully.

24.6.2 Manual Methods for Bacteriological Examination of the Urine Sample for Diagnosis of Urinary Tract Infection (UTI) Includes Following Steps

1. Physical examination.
2. A definitive urine culture.
3. Screening test for significant bacteriuria by microscopic examination, and quantitative assessment.
4. Demonstration of antibody coating of bacteria present in the urinary sediment using fluorescein dye conjugated antihuman gamma globulin (in case advised).
5. A blood culture for UTI patients showing symptoms of systemic illness (if advised).
6. Antibiotic sensitivity test of isolated organisms.

24.6.2.1 Materials Required

- Urine specimen, properly labeled and properly transported.
- Microscope, glass slides, coverslips.

- Culture plates—MacConkey agar, blood agar and Müller-Hinton (MH) agar.
- Calibrated inoculating loop.
- Antibiotic discs.

24.6.2.2 Procedure

	Performance of tests	*Remarks*
Day 1	**Culture:** With a calibrated sterilized loop (holding 0.01 ml or 0.001 ml of urine), aseptically inoculate one MacConkey agar plate and one blood agar plate by streak plate method to obtain isolated colonies. Incubate the plates at 37°C overnight.	May give a preliminary report on the basis of microscopic examination
	Physical examination: Examine the urine sample macroscopically for presence of cloudiness, odour (e.g. aromatic odour indicates *Pseudomonas* infection, ammoniacal odour indicates *Proteus* infection).	
	Microscopic examination: Examine the un-spun urine under the high power field (hpf) of the microscope for epithelial cells and WBC and a gram stained smear under oil immersion objective to assess the suitability of urine sample for culture. More than 10 WBC per high power field (hpf) in un-spun urine represents pyuria. More than 5–10 epithelial cells per hpf usually indicates contamination. In the gram stained smear, 1 or more bacteria per oil immersion field indicates an approximate bacterial number of 10^5 per ml. Presence of 1 or more leukocytes per oil immersion field suggests UTI.	
	Primary sensitivity test in case there is significant bacteruria, put up a primary antibiotic sensitivity test on MH agar using surface swabbing by soaking a sterile swab in the urine sample and incubate overnight.	
Day 2	- Examine the blood agar plate and MacConkey agar plate for growth and colony characteristic of the organisms. Count approximate number of colonies. - Inoculate isolated colonies in liquid medium for further identification of the organism by biochemical tests and for putting up the antibiotic sensitivity test. - Check the primary sensitivity plate for antibiotic sensitivity.	May give a presumptive report
Day 3	- If no growth appears in 24, report "No Growth". - For urine sample growing more than 2 species of bacteria with a count of less than or equal to 10^4 bacteria per ml of urine, report mixed growth of Gram-positive and/or Gram-negative bacteria-probably contaminants. - In case of mixed growth with count of 10^3 to 10^4 bacteria/ml or growth of three or more species of organism having a viable count of more than or equal to 10^4 bacteria/ml, report only the viable count without processing the culture for species identification and antibiotic sensitivity test. - In case of growth of a single species or two species of organisms with a bacterial count of more than 10^5 bacteria/ml, report the viable count, name(s) of the isolate(s) and the antibiotic sensitivity of each isolate.	Give the final report

24.6.2.3 Laboratory Record of Urine Culture

Maintain a record of urine samples processed by you

Date	Result	In case of positive bacteriuria		Teacher's signature
		Organism isolated	Antibiotic sensitivity	

Processing of Fecal Sample for Culture and Sensitivity

25.1 AIM

To educate the students the importance of stool as a specimen for the diagnosis of intestinal infections and the correct procedure for culture and sensitivity of the causative organism to reach a confirmatory diagnosis.

25.2 LEARNING OUTCOME

Students learn to perform the stool culture efficiently.

25.3 PURPOSE

Stool culture is indicated for diagnosis of diarrheal diseases, cholera, dysentery and food poisoning associated with gastrointestinal tract (Fig. 25.1).

25.4 PATHOGENIC AND COMMENSAL ORGANISMS ISOLATED FROM STOOL

Pathogens	Commensals
Shigella, Vibrio cholerae, Vibrio parahaemolyticus, Mycobacterium tuberculosis, enteropathogenic *Escherichia coli, Campylobacter, Clostridium perfringens, Clostridium botulinum, Staphylococcus, Bacillus, Salmonella, Yersinia, etc.*	Commensals are present in stool in very high numbers. Organisms are lactobacillus, Enterobacteriaceae, yeast, anaerobic bacteria, bacteroides, etc.

25.5 COLLECTION OF SPECIMEN

General guidelines for diagnosis of bacterial infection in the gastrointestinal tract are as under:

25.5.1 Specimen

A stool specimen is always preferred rather than a rectal swab.

Collection of a stool specimen
- Collect the specimen at an early stage of illness and prior to any antimicrobial treatment.
- Do not collect the specimen from bedpan.
- Ensure that the stool specimen is not contaminated with urine.
- Collect the sample in a wide mouth disposable container.
- If possible, receive more than one specimen on different days.

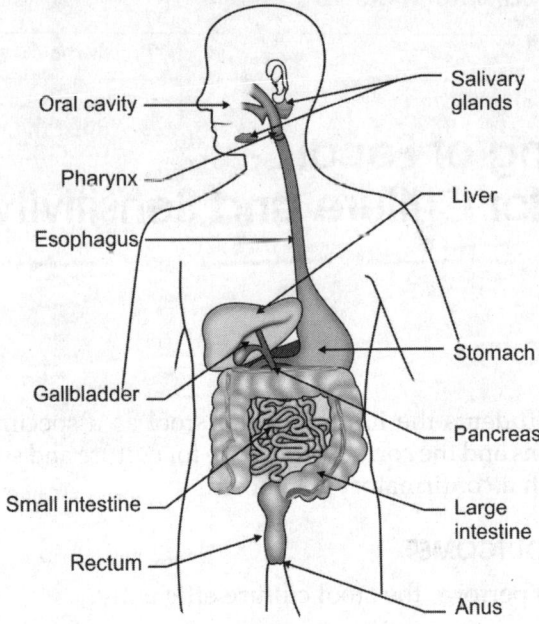

Fig. 25.1: Gastrointestinal tract

- 1 – 2 g quantity is sufficient.
- Stool specimen must be received within 1–2 hours of passage.

25.5.2 Collection of Rectal Swab

1. Insert swab at least 2.5 cm beyond the anal sphincter for reaching the rectum.
2. Rotate the swab once before withdrawing.
3. Place the swab in a suitable transport medium for sending to the laboratory.

25.6 MEDIA FOR TRANSPORT AND/OR PROCESSING OF FECAL SPECIMEN/RECTAL SWAB

25.6.1 Cary Blair Transport Medium

Composition	Preparation
• Sodium chloride: 5.00 gm/lit. • Sodium thioglycollate:1.50 gm/lit. • Disodium hydrogen phosphate:1.1gm/lit. Agar 5.00g/litre • 1% calcium chloride solution: 0.1 gm in 10 ml distilled water • pH at 25°C:8.0 ± 0.5 Storage: Store between 8°C and 25°C.	1. Add ingredients to distilled/deionized water. 2. Mix thoroughly.Bring volume to 1.0 liter. 3. Gently heat until boiling. 4. Cool to 50°C and add 9.0 ml of 1% calcium chloride solution. 5. Adjust pH to 8.4. 6. Dispense in 9 ml screw capped bottles in 7 ml portions. 7. Sterilize under free steam for 15 minutes. 8. Cool and tighten the cap of the bottle.

25.6.2 Stuart's Transport Medium

Composition	Preparation
A. Anaerobic salt solution • Thioglycollic acid 2 ml. • 1N sodium hydroxide 12–15 ml. • 20% sodium glycerol phosphate solution in chlorine free distilled water 100 ml. • 1% calcium chloride in chlorine free distilled water 20 ml. • Chlorine free distilled water 900 ml pH 7.2 **B. Agar solution** 6 g agar in 1000 ml chlorine free distilled water, dissolved by steaming. **C. Methylene blue solution** 0.1% methylene blue solution in chlorine free distilled water. **Complete medium** A. Anaerobic salt solution -900 ml. B. Agar solution -1000 ml. C. Methylene blue solution -4 ml.	1. Mix the solutions A,B and C. 2. Adjust the pH to 7.3–7.4 3. Distribute in bottles. 4. Sterilize at 121°C for 15 minutes. Medium should be colourless when cooled.

25.6.3 Selenite F broth, used for Isolation and Cultivation of *Salmonella* Species from Faeces, Dairy Products and other Specimens

Composition	Preparation
• Pancreatic digest of casein: 5.00 gm/litre • Disodium hydrogen phosphate: 3.00 gm/litre • Lactose: 4.00 gm/litre • Potassium dihydrogen phosphate: 7.00 gm/litre • Sodium selenite: 4 g/litre pH at 25°C: 7.0 ± 0.2 Storage: Store between 8 and 25°C.	1. Add all ingredients to distilled/deionized water. 2. Bring the volume to 1.0 litre. 3. Gently heat and bring to boiling. Dispense in tubes. 4. Sterilize in boiling water bath or at 0 psi pressure at 100°C for 10 minutes.

25.6.4 *Campylobacter* Blood Agar (for *Campylobacter*)

Composition	Preparation
***Campylobacter* blood agar base** • Beef extract 5 g • Peptone 5 g • Sodium chloride 2.5 g • Agar 7.5 g • Water 500 ml **Antimicrobic supplements** • Cycloheximide 50 mg • Rifampicin 5 mg • Trimetoprim 5 mg • Polymyxin B 2500 units • pH 7.5–7.7 **Lysed sterile horse blood 25 ml**	1. Suspend the ingredients in 500 ml distilled water. 2. Heat to boiling. 3. Sterilize by autoclaving at 121°C for 15 minutes. 4. Cool to 50°C. 5. Add the antimicrobic supplements together with 25 ml of lysed sterile horse blood. 6. Mix well and immediately distribute in sterile petridishes. 7. Store at 4°C.

25.6.5 Venkataraman-Ramakrishnan Medium (for *V. cholerae*)

(10 ml medium is used for 1–3 ml of stool sample)

Composition	Preparation
Stock solution Boric acid (H₃BO₃) 12.405 g Potassium chloride 14.912 g Distilled water 1 litre **Working solution (1 litre)** M/5 sodium hydroxide 133.5 ml/250 ml of stock solution Dried sea salt/common salt 20 g pH 9.2	1. **Stock solution** Dissolve boric acid and potassium chloride in 800 ml of hot distilled water, cool and make up the volume to 1 litre. 2. **Working solution** Add 20 g of salt to the mixture of 250 ml of stock solution and 133.5 ml of M/5 NaOH. • Make up the volume to 1 litre with distilled water. • Distribute in 10 ml quantities in 28 ml screw capped bottles. Sterilize by autoclaving at 15 lbs pressure for 15 mins.

25.7 PROCEDURE

	Performance of tests	Remarks
Day 1	Take the specimen with as much mucus as possible. **Macroscopic examination:** Examine macroscopically for consistency of the sample, foreign bodies, adult worms, tape worm segments, blood and for special character like rice water stool. **Microscopic examination:** Examine wet film preparation for presence of leukocytes (indicating infection by entero-invasive bacteria), movement of the organisms like a shoal of fish, etc. Examine Gram stained smear for *Staph. aureus* and *Candida*. **Culture** Inoculate in • Medium for selective detection of *Salmonella*, *Shigella*, *Vibrio* or other gram negative bacillary pathogens (MacConkey or XLD medium). • BAP for detection of *Staphylococcus aureus* and yeast. • An enrichment broth, e.g. selenite broth, tetrathionate broth for detection of small number of *Salmonella*. • Inoculate alkaline peptone water/V.R medium for *Vibrio*. • *Campylobacter* blood agar plate for *Campylobacter*. • Incubate at 37°C for overnight.	May give a preliminary report based on macro-scopic and microscopic examination.
Day 2	1. Check BAP for over growth of *Staphylococcus*/yeast. 2. Put up antibiotic sensitivity test for *Staphylococcus*, if there is overgrowth of *Staphylococcus*. 3. Check *Campylobacter* BAP for growth of *Campylobacter*. 4. Check the MacConkey/XLD plates for NLF colonies. Check suspicious colonies with oxidase test since unusual cases of diarrhoea includes *Vibrio parahaemolyticus* and *Aeromonus* species. 5. Perform cholera red test	

(Contd.)

(Contd.)

	Performance of tests	Remarks
	6. Reject LF colonies except for toxin check for *Escherichia* species. 7. Inoculate TSI slants with pure culture of NLF. 8. Put up biochemical tests for H$_2$S production, motility and slide agglutination for further confirmation. 9. Subculture from the selenite broth for detection of Gram-negative bacillary pathogens on XLD medium.	
Day 3	Read the biochemical tests of pure culture. If necessary, do the slide agglutination test. Examine subculture plates and put up biochemical tests with additional colonies, if necessary. Put up the sensitivity tests, if required.	Send a final report in case no suspicious colony is found on subculture
Day 4	Identify the suspicious colony found on subculture from broth culture.	Send a final report

25.8 LABORATORY RECORD OF STOOL CULTURE

Maintain a record of stool culture done by you.

Date	Organism isolated	Antibiotic sensitivity	Teacher's signature

Processing of Pus Sample for Culture and Sensitivity

26.1 AIM

To educate the students the importance of pus culture in the diagnosis of wound infection.

26.2 LEARNING OUTCOME

Students learn the method of collection of pus from the wound, abscess and to perform the pus culture efficiently.

26.3 PURPOSE

Pus culture is indicated for diagnosis of infections of wound, abscess, burns and sinuses caused by various aerobic and anaerobic bacteria.

Schematic diagram of the skin with pus formation is shown in Fig. 26.1.

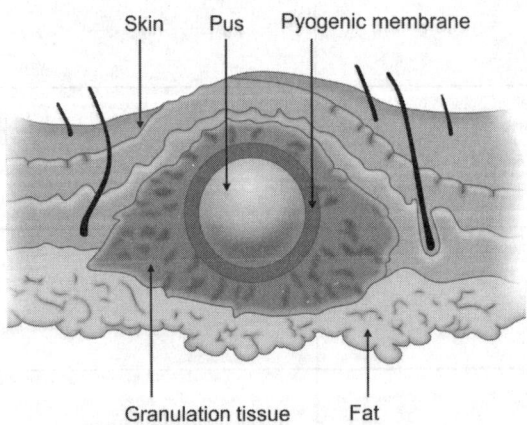

Fig. 26.1: Schematic diagram of skin with pus formation

26.4 PATHOGENS AND COMMENSAL ORGANISMS FOUND IN PUS CULTURE

Pathogens	Commensal
Pseudomonas, Staphylococcus aureus, Streptococcus pyogenes, Proteus, Escherichia coli, Klebsiella, Clostridium, etc.	Skin commensals, Streptococcus viridians, Staphylococcus albus, Diphtheroids, aerobic spore bearers, yeast, etc.

26.5 COLLECTION OF SPECIMEN

a. **From wound incision or wound drainage:** Collect up to 1 ml of pus with sterile capillary or from the drainage tube. Transfer to a sterile container and label.

b. **From wound without drainage:** Swab the area around the wound with 70% alcohol. Aspirate with needle and syringe. Cleanse rubber stopper of vial containing anaerobic transport medium with alcohol; allow to dry 1 min before inoculating; push needle through septum and inject all abscess material on top of agar. If a swab must be used, pass the swab deep into the base of the infected site to collect the specimen. Collect minimum two samples. Immerse the swabs in the transport medium. Maintain at room temperature. Send to the laboratory within 30 minutes of collection.

26.6 PROCESSING OF SAMPLE

	Performance of tests	*Remarks*
Day 1	**Macroscopic examination**—Green/bluish green colour indicates *Pseudomonas* infection **Microscopic examination**—Perform gram staining. **Culture**—inoculate on BAP, CAP. MAP and in thioglycollate broth.	Give a preliminary report of Gram staining
Day 2	1. Examine the plates. Identify the organisms by their colony characteristics. 2. Put up biochemical tests. 3. Subculture from thioglycollate broth for 3. Identification of anaerobic pathogen 4. Put up antibiotic sensitivity test	
Day 3 subsequent days	Identify the isolate. Read the sensitivity plates.	Give final report with the name of the isolate and anti-biotic sensitivity

26.7 LABORATORY RECORD

Maintain a record for pus samples processed by you for culture and sensitivity.

Date	*Results of macroscopic and microscopic examination*	*Organism isolated*	*Antimicrobial sensitivity*	*Teacher's signature*

27

Processing of Throat Swab and Nasopharyngeal Swab Samples for Culture and Sensitivity

27.1 AIM

To educate the students the importance of throat swab and nasopharyngeal swab as specimens for diagnosis of upper respiratory tract infection, correct procedures for collection and culture of these swabs and sensitivity to reach a confirmatory diagnosis.

27.2 LEARNING OUTCOME

Students learn to perform throat swab culture and nasopharyngeal swab culture efficiently.

Human respiratory tract is broadly divided into two parts: upper respiratory tract consisting of nasal cavity, pharynx and larynx and lower respiratory tract consisting of trachea, bronchi and lungs (Fig. 27.1).

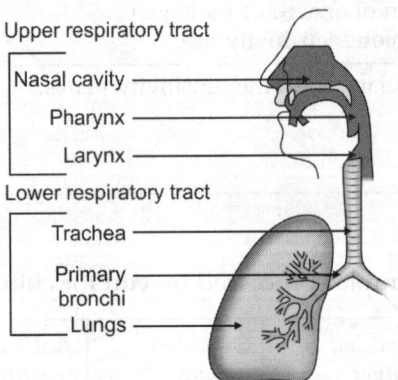

Upper respiratory tract
- Nasal cavity
- Pharynx
- Larynx

Lower respiratory tract
- Trachea
- Primary bronchi
- Lungs

Fig. 27.1: Human respiratory tract

27.3 PURPOSE

Throat swab and nasopharyngeal swab are used as specimens related to upper respiratory tract infection and are used for following purposes:

- To diagnose sore throat and other infections in the upper respiratory tract generally caused by *Bordetella pertussis* or *Corynebacterium diphtheriae, and* streptococcal infections
- To identify carriers of *Staphylococcus aureus, Streptococcus pneumoniae,* and *Neisseria meningitides* that may transmit these organisms via nasal secretions to others organs/places resulting in serious infections, e.g. *Streptococcus pneumoniae* can cause pneumonia and septicemia and *N. meningitides* can cause outbreaks of meningitis.

27.4 COMMENSALS AND PATHOGENS ISOLATED FROM UPPER RESPIRATORY TRACT

Pathogens	*Commensals*
Bordetella pertussis, Corynebacterium diphtheriae, Staphylococcus aureus, Streptococcus pyogenes, *Neisseria meningitides, Chlamydia trachomatis,* group A beta-hemolytic streptococci, *Neisseria gonorrhoeae, etc.*	*Strept.viridans, Diphtheroids, Aerobic spore bearers, Haemophilus influenzae, Streptococcus pneumoniae, Candida albicans* present in small number, etc.
Haemophilus influenzae, Streptococcus pneumoniae, Candida albicans, if present in very large number.	

In most cases of upper respiratory tract infections, a throat culture is more appropriate than a nasopharyngeal culture. However, the nasopharyngeal culture should be used in cases where throat cultures are difficult to obtain or to detect the carrier status especially for meningococcal disease.

27.5 COLLECTION OF SPECIMEN

27.5.1 Collection of Throat Swab (Fig. 27.2A)

1. Check the expiry date of the transport media (generally Stuart or Amies transport medium) and the swab.
2. Make the patient sit in a well-lit area so that his/her posterior mouth cavity is clearly visible.
3. Ask the patient to bend back his/her head and gently depress the tongue with a tongue depressor.
4. Rub the posterior pharynx and the tonsillar area with the swab specifically targeting the inflamed area, if any, without touching the lateral walls of the mouth cavity or the tongue. Sample the exudate present, if any.
5. Place the swab in the transport tube. Cap the tube to avoid contamination of the specimen.
6. Label the specimen and send to the laboratory.

27.5.2 Collection of Nasopharyngeal Swab (Fig. 27.2B)

Nasopharynx is the back wall of the nasal cavity where it meets the throat (Fig. 27.2B). Nasopharyngeal swabs are mostly used to collect samples from neonates or young children who have an upper respiratory infection.

Procedure for Collection of Nasopharyngeal Swab

Use personal protective equipment: wear a surgical mask and disposable gloves.

1. Wash hands thoroughly with soap and water or alcohol based hand gel before and after the procedure.
2. Gently clean out visible nasal mucus and the nostril with a cotton swab.
3. Use a flexible fine shafted aluminum swab with rayon or calcium alginate tip.
4. Prior to insertion, measure the distance from the corner of the nose to the front of the ear and insert the shaft only half this length.

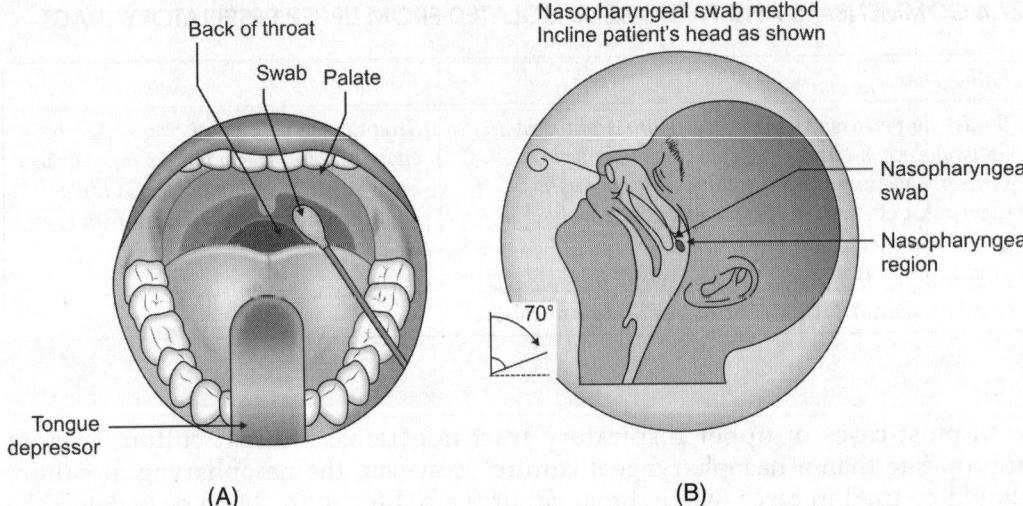

Fig. 27.2: Collection of specimens for upper respiratory tract infection: (A) throat swab (B) nasopharyngeal swab

5. Make the patient comfortable. Slightly tilt the patient's head back to straighten the light path from the front of the nose to the nasopharynx to make insertion of the swab easier.
6. Insert the swab gently along the medial part of the septum, along the floor of the nose, until it reaches the posterior part.
7. Allow the swab to sit in place for 5–10 seconds.
8. Rotate the swab several times to dislodge the columnar epithelial cells.
9. Withdraw the swab and place it in the collection tube.
10. Refrigerate immediately.
11. Remove gloves. Wash hands.
12. Attach completed requisition. Transport specimen to the laboratory.

27.6 STORAGE

In case there is a delay in processing the specimen, keep the sample refrigerated at 4°C for up to 72 hours. For bacterial culture, place the swab in Stuart's transport medium.

27.7 PROCESSING OF SPECIMEN

	Performance of tests	*Remarks*
Day 1	In case the swabs have been collected in the laboratory, collect the swabs in duplicate. Use **one swab for microscopic examination**, if indicated. • Perform Gram staining to indicate *Candida*, *Corynebacteria*, Meningococi and Vincent's organisms • Perform Albert staining for diphtheria bacilli **Culture**: Based on the requisition, use the swab for direct streak plating or subculture from transport medium on, • Sheep BAP, (for most of the pathogens including *Streptococcus* and *Staphylococcus*).	Give preliminary report in case of suspected diphtheria case

(Contd.)

(Contd.)

	Performance of tests	Remarks
	• CAP(for *Haemophilus*) in case of sore throat and epiglottitis. • MacConkey plate for Gram-negative bacilli (in case of otitis media and sinusitis). • On Loefller's media, if diphtheria is suspected. • Thioglycollate media in case of foul smelling exudate, for anaerobic organisms. • Bordet Gengou medium for suspected *Bordetella* infection. Incubate the cultures at 35°C in air at high humidity.	
Day 2	1. Make pure culture. 2. Identify the organism by colony characteristics and biochemical reactions. Preliminary identification of the organism can be made from catalase, coagulase, urease, nitrate reduction, sucrose fermentation tests and characteristic colonial morphology. 3. Put up antibiotic sensitivity test.	For pathogens other than diphtheria bacilli, give the final report along with the antibiotic sensitivity
Day 3	After 48 hours discard plates showing no growth of suspected pathogens. Retain plates for *C. diphtheriae* or *B. pertussis*, if suspected, for 6–7 days.	

27.8 LABORATORY RECORD

Perform throat swab and nasopharyngeal swab culture and record your observations.

Date	Organism isolated	Antimicrobial sensitivity	Teacher's signature

Processing of Sputum Sample for Culture and Sensitivity

28.1 AIM

To educate the students the importance of sputum as a specimen for the diagnosis of lower respiratory tract infection and correct procedure to be adopted for culture of sputum and sensitivity to reach a confirmatory diagnosis.

28.2 LEARNING OUTCOME

Students learn the importance the collection of a true sputum sample and to perform the sputum culture efficiently.

28.3 PURPOSE

Sputum culture is indicated whenever bacterial (including mycobacterial) infection or fungal infection is suspected in the lower respiratory tract (Fig. 27.1).

28.4 PATHOGENS AND CONTAMINANTS FOUND IN SPUTUM

Pathogens	Contaminants
Staphylococcus aureus, Klebsiella, Neisseria meningitides, group A beta-hemolytic Streptococci, Haemophilus influenzae, Streptococcus pneumoniae, Candida albicans, Mycobacterium tuberculosis, etc.	All commensals of upper respiratory tract

28.5 COLLECTION OF SPUTUM

Sputum must represent the true pulmonary expectoration and not the saliva or the secretion from nose or pharynx. Morning sputum should be collected in a wide mouth container. Correct method of sputum collection is shown in Fig. 28.1.

- Advise the patient to brush his/her teeth and rinse the mouth to reduce contamination with the bacteria of the mouth cavity.
- Give the patient a wide mouth sputum container made up of clear, thin, leak proof and unbreakable material. Show the patient how to open and close the container.
- Tell the person to take a standing position and breath in and out three times.
- Tell the person to take a deep breath filling his/her lungs, to empty the lungs in one breath coughing as hard as possible, to bring the wide mouth container close to his/her mouth and to spit the sputum in the container.
- Make sure that the sputum is thick, purulent and sufficient in amount (2–3 ml).
- Label the container.

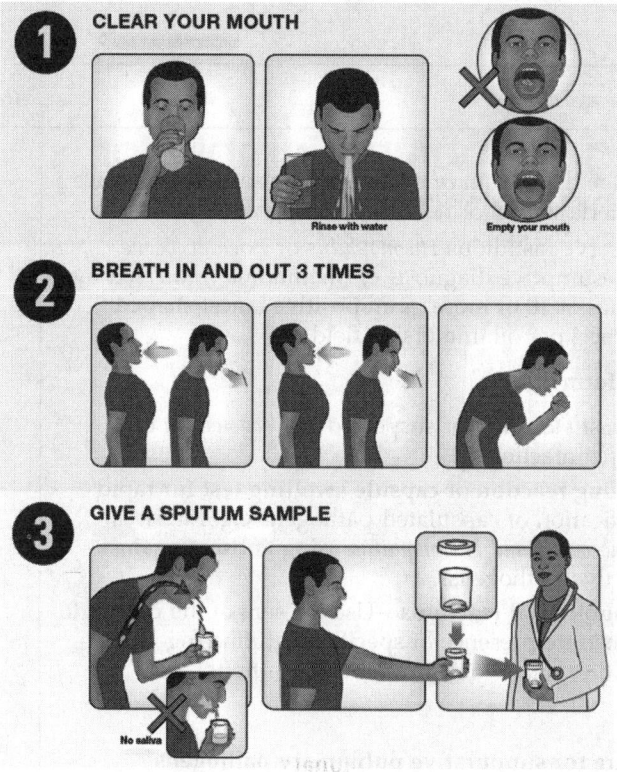

Fig. 28.1: Correct method of sputum collection

28.6 PROCESSING OF THE SPUTUM

Sputum should be processed within 1 hour of collection.

	Performance of tests	Remarks
Day 1	**1. Macroscopic examination** Note the colour, odour and consistency, presence of blood, if any. A clear specimen indicates saliva. A thick, tenacious sputum suggests infection by *Klebsiella pneumoniae*, a foul odour suggests infection by anaerobic organism. **2. Microscopic examination** **(a) Examine wet film preparation for** • Presence of parasitic eggs, fungus, etc. • **Leukocyte and macrophages** (Less than 10 epithelial cells/low power field and more than 25 leukocytes and alveolar macrophages per low power field reflects a true sputum sample). **(b) Examine following stained preparations** **Do Gram stain**	Give a report on acid fast staining and immunological reactions

(Contd.)

(Contd.)

Performance of tests	*Remarks*
• To judge the adequacy of the sputum sample (presence of bacteria within or near the neutrophils). • To observe fastidious *Haemophilus* or *Pneumococcus*. • For presumptive diagnosis of pneumonia (indicated by presence of 10 or more gram positive lancet shaped diplococci per oil immersion field). **Also perform** • **Acid fast staining** for suspected *Mycobacterium* or *Nocardia* infection. • **Quellung reaction or capsule swelling test for** rapid identification of capsulated pathogens e.g. *Klebsiella, Pneumococcus and Haemophilus* using antisera against respective pathogens. • **Immunological reactions**—Use the sera of the patient to demonstrate presence of specific agglutinating antibodies or for immunostaining methods. **3. Culture** **A. Culture for suppurative pulmonary pathogens** Select a floccule or purulent portion of the sputum and inoculate directly into each of a BAP, CAP and MacConkey agar plate (MAP). **Or** Homogenise the sputum sample with pancreatin and inoculate on BAP, CAP or MAP. **Or** With two sterile inoculating loop wash a purulent portion in sterile water three times. Then inoculate on BAP, CAP and MAP. If specifically indicated, also inoculate mannitol salt agar, Sabouraud's agar and thioglycollate broth. **B. Culture for non-suppurative pulmonary pathogens** *Mycobacterium tuberculosis* Concentrate the sputum sample by Petroff's method. Take equal volume of sputum and 4% NaOH in a sterile sealable container, incubate at room temperature for 15 to 20 minutes mixing regularly at intervals of 5 minutes. Centrifuge the mixture at 3000–4000 rpm for less than 10 minutes. Discard the supernatant in a disinfectant solution. Neutralize the sediment with 8% hydrochloric acid with phenol red as indicator. Use the sediment for acid fast staining and inoculate at least three bottles of Lowenstein Jensen media.	

(Contd.)

	Performance of tests	*Remarks*
	Bordetella pertussis Inoculate on Bordet-Gengue medium containing penicillin. Use one nasopharyngeal swab also for inoculation. **Virus – Sputum or throat washing may be cultured** **4. Incubate at 35°C overnight** (for *Mycobacterium*, incubation period is 3 weeks)	
Day 2	**Examine the growth and colony characteristics** • *S. pneumoniae* appear as small, gray, moist (sometimes mucoid), watery colonies on CAP with a surrounding green zone of α-hemolysis on BAP. After 24–48 hours incubation, the colonies become flattened, and the central portion becomes depressed. There is a zone of inhibition around optochin disc, if placed in the BAP. • *H. influenza* appear as large, colorless-to-gray, opaque colonies on a CAP. No discoloration of the medium is apparent. Encapsulated strains appear more mucoidal than non-encapsulated strains, which appear as smaller compact gray colonies. • Brittle, dry, gray white colonies on both BAP and CAP with a positive oxidase test indicates *Branhamella catarrhalis.* • *Staphylococcus aureus* grow as golden yellow, medium size colonies with complete hemolysis on BAP. Mannitol fermentation test and coagulase tests are positive. • Whitish, round, matt colonies may be that of *Candida albicans* • On MAP, enteric organisms grow. Identify them by routine methods. Put up additional biochemical test, if required. Based on the organism isolated, put up antibiotic sensitivity test on MH agar for enteric organisms and *Staphylococcus*, on CAP for *Haemophilus* and on lysed BAP for rest of the isolates.	Give a preliminary report on growth of presumptive organism(s) as under: Name of the isolate with number of colonies as: (i) a few colonies, (ii) a light growth, (iii) a moderately heavy growth or (iv) a heavy growth.
Day 3	Examine the antibiotic sensitivity plates	Give complete report with antibiotic sensitivity

28.7 LABORATORY RECORD

Perform sputum culture. Record your observations.

Date	Results of macroscopic, microscopic and immunological examination	Name of the organism isolated	Antimicrobial sensitivity	Teacher's signature

Processing of Blood Sample for Culture and Sensitivity

29.1 AIM

To educate the students the importance of blood culture in the diagnosis of septicemia (spread of infection in the blood) and correct procedure for collection, culture and sensitivity of blood in order to reach a confirmatory diagnosis.

29.2 LEARNING OUTCOME

Students learn to collect blood sample and perform the blood culture efficiently.

29.3 PURPOSE

Blood culture is indicated whenever bacterial, fungal, or mycobacterial sepsis is suspected, with the possible exception of minor mucocutaneous infections or of lower urinary tract infections.

29.4 PATHOGENS ISOLATED FROM BLOOD

Pathogens	Commensal
Streptococcus, Staphylococcus, Pseudomonas, Salmonella, Candida, Escherichia coli, Pneumococcus, fungus, anaerobic organisms, any organism that can invade bloodstream from infections in other organs	None

29.5 GENERAL GUIDELINES OR COLLECTION OF BLOOD FOR BLOOD CULTURE

- Collect blood before starting antibiotic therapy.
- Collect blood during the early stages of disease.
- Collect blood when the patient is having high temperature.
- Skin antisepsis is extremely important at the time of collection of sample.
- Collect less quantity of blood from children.
- For bacterial or fungal sepsis, collect two specimens per patient by separate venipuncture.
- In case of bacterial endocarditis, as there is intermittent bacteria release, collect maximum four sets of blood specimens in one 24 hours period. If all four sets are negative after 24 hours and sepsis is still suspected, more cultures may be collected.
- Infants and small children: Two blood cultures usually are sufficient (one may suffice in the neonate).
- Keep two blood culture bottles, (ratio of specimen:medium shall be 1:10) one for aerobic organisms (e.g. tryptic soya broth with SPS) and another for anaerobic organisms (e.g. thioglycollate broth) ready for immediate inoculation.

29.6 PROCEDURE FOR BLOOD COLLECTION (VENIPUNCTURE USING NEEDLE AND SYRINGE) (Fig. 29.1)

1. Wash hands and wear gloves.
2. Apply a tourniquet and palpate arm of the patient for suitable vein.
3. Clean the patient's skin by scrubbing with 70% alcohol swab up and down and side-to-side for 30 seconds. Allow to air dry.
4. Prepare the blood culture bottle(s) having media volume ten times the volume of the specimens (1: 10 dilution).
5. Do not touch the venipuncture site.
6. Place needle on syringe. For routine blood cultures, collect appropriate volume of blood (if pediatric patient, volume of blood is determined by patient's weight).
7. Remove needle and apply pressure to venipuncture site.
8. Without allowing needle to become potentially contaminated, or blood getting clotted in the syringe, place syringe directly into one blood culture bottle. For routine cultures, distribute equal volume of blood into each bottle with a final ratio of medium: blood =10:1, inoculate anaerobic culture medium also.

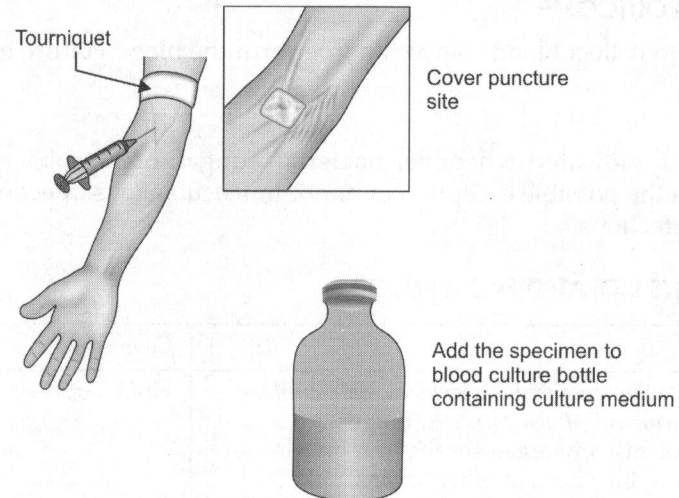

Tourniquet

Cover puncture site

Add the specimen to blood culture bottle containing culture medium

Fig. 29.1: Collection of blood sample for culture

29.7 CULTURE MEDIA USED FOR BLOOD CULTURE

29.7.1 Trypticase Soya Broth (TSB)

Sodium polyanethol sulfonate (SPS) or sodium amylosulfate (SAS) may be added to one of the culture bottles for antagonizing host defense mechanism.

Composition	Preparation
• Tryptone (pancreatic digest of casein) 17.0 g • Soytone (peptic digest of soybean meal) 3.0 g • Glucose (dextrose) 2.5 g • Sodium chloride 5.0 g • Dipotassium hydrogen phosphate 2.5 g • Distilled water 1 litre, pH 7.3 ± 0.2	1. Dissolve the ingredients in distilled water. 2. Distribute in screw capped bottles in 90 ml quantities (for 10 ml blood). 3. Sterilize by autoclaving at 8 lbs for 30 minutes.

29.7.2 Thioglycollate Broth

Composition	Preparation
• L-cystine 0.5 g • Agar (granulated) 0.75 g • Sodium chloride 2.5 g • Dextrose 5 g • Yeast extract 5 g • Tryptone 15 g • Sodium thioglycollate or thioglycollic acid 0.5 g • Resazurin sodium (1:1000 solution) fresh 1 ml • Distilled water 1 litre	1. Weigh the ingredients. 2. Mix L-cystine, NaCl, dextrose, yeast extract, and tryptone with 1 liter water. 3. Heat in Arnold steamer or in a water bath until ingredients are dissolved. 4. Dissolve sodium thioglycollate or thioglycollic acid in solution. 5. Adjust pH so that value after sterilization is 7.1 ± 0.2. 6. Add sodium resazurin solution, mix. 7. Dispense in blood culture bottles in 90 ml quantities (for 10 ml blood) 8. Sterilise by autoclaving for 15–20 min at 121°C. 9. Store in the dark at room temperature.

29.8 PROCESSING BLOOD SPECIMENS

	Performance of tests	Remarks
Day 1	Transport the inoculated blood culture bottle to the laboratory immediately after collection for incubation at 35–37°C with ~5% CO_2 (or in a candle-jar) and sub-culture. In case immediate transport to the laboratory is not possible, keep the inoculated bottle in an incubator at 35–37°C with approximate 5% carbon dioxide till transport is possible.	
Day 2	Examine the blood culture broth, every day for up to 7 days. In case of any turbidity, lysis of erythrocytes, growth of apparent colonies and gas production, immediately subculture on plates and perform Gram staining from the blood culture. Perform blind subcultures on BAP and CAP after 18 hours incubation in following manner: • Disinfect the rubber septum of the blood culture bottle (that shows turbidity) with a 70% alcohol swab. Alternatively, if the blood culture bottle has a screw-cap, open the bottle and remove the fluid using sterile technique (i.e. flaming the bottle mouth upon opening and closing the cap). • Swirl the blood culture bottle to mix the contents. Aseptically aspirate 1 ml with a sterile syringe and needle from the blood culture bottle and transfer 0.5 ml to a BAP, 0.5 ml to a CAP and 0.5 ml to a MacConkey medium. Streak the plates for isolation, incubate at 35–37°C with ~5% CO_2 (or in a candle-jar), and examine daily for up to 72 hours.	
Day 3 and subsequent days	Inspect the isolates for purity of growth by looking at colony morphology before any testing is performed. If any contamination is seen, cultures should be re-streaked to ensure purity prior to testing.	Give final report

Total period of incubation of a routine blood culture is 5 days. However, on specific request of the physician, cultures are kept and inspected daily for 2–4 weeks.

Once pure bacterial growth has been confirmed by subculture from blood culture bottle, dispose the bottle following to proper safety procedures.

29.9 AUTOMATED METHOD

In the Biomerieux BacT/AlerT 3D culture system, production of carbon dioxide by the organisms is detected colourimetrically. Culture bottles are constantly agitated and read at ten minutes intervals. Carbon dioxide produced by the organisms lowers the pH of the medium. Change in the colour of the medium is compiled in a computer compiler and report generated.

29.10 LABORATORY RECORDS

Perform blood culture and record your findings

Date	Organism isolated	Anti-microbial sensitivity report	Teacher's signature

Processing of Cerebrospinal Fluid Sample for Culture and Sensitivity

30.1 AIM

To educate the students the importance of CSF culture in the diagnosis of meningitis, and correct procedure for CSF collection, culture and sensitivity for reaching a confirmatory diagnosis.

30.2 LEARNING OUTCOME

Students learn to perform the CSF culture efficiently.

30.3 PURPOSE

Cerebrospinal fluid is the specimen for diagnosis of meningitis, i.e. infection in the meninges. A cerebrospinal fluid (CSF) culture is a laboratory procedure to look for bacteria and fungi in the normally clear fluid that surrounds the brain and spinal cord.

Pathogens	Commensal
Haemophilus, Neisseria, Pneumococcus, Brucella, Salmonella, Mycobacterium tuberculosis, Leptospira, Candida albicans, Nocardia, Cryptococcus, Histoplasma and other organisms	None

30.4 CSF COLLECTION

Cerebrospinal fluid (CSF) is generally collected by lumbar puncture (Fig. 30.1)

- Collect CSF before starting antibiotic therapy.
- Advise the patient to lie on his or her side, with knees pulled up toward the chest, and chin tucked downward. In case the collection is done with the person sitting up, he/she must bend forward.
- After the back is cleaned with 70% alcohol, inject a local anesthetic agent into the lower spine.
- Insert a spinal needle 22G/3.5 (for adults)/23G/2.5 (for children) into the lower back area between L 3 and L 4 (Fig. 30.1).
- Once the needle is properly positioned, measure the CSF pressure and collect a sample(3–4 ml, minimum 1 ml) in a fresh sterile fresh screw capped container.
- Remove the needle, clean the area and place a bandage over the needle site. The person may lie down for a short time after CSF collection.

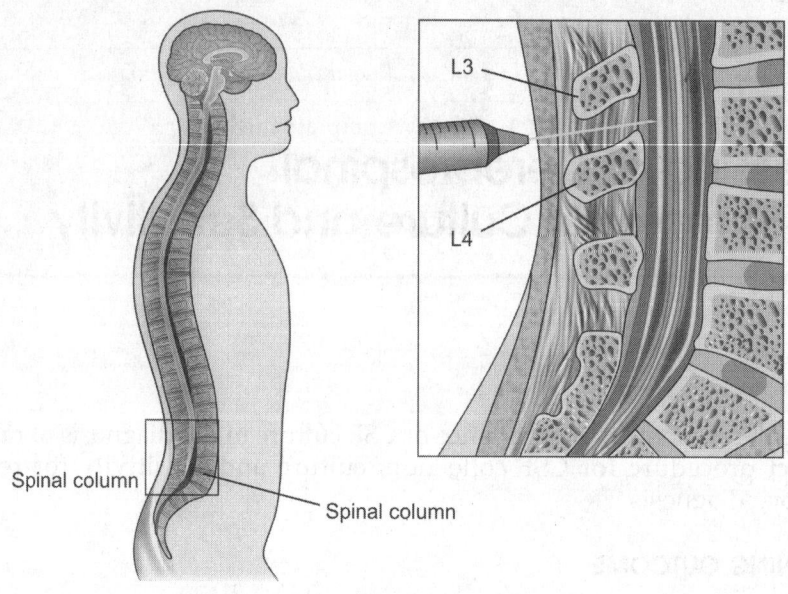

Fig. 30.1: Collection of cerebrospinal fluid

30.5 TRANSPORT

Do not delay transport of CSF. In case delay is unavoidable, keep the specimen at 37°C or use a transport medium, e.g. biphasic trans-isolate medium for transport.

30.6 PREPARATION OF CULTURE MEDIUM

30.6.1 Preparation of Trans-isolate (T-I) Medium

Ingredient	Preparation of the medium
a. **Diluents for solid and liquid phases:** • 0.1M 3-N-morpholino propanesulfonic acid (MOPS) buffer 20.93 g • Distilled water up to 1000 ml after adjusting to pH 7.2 with sodium hydroxide b. **Solid phase:** • Activated charcoal 2.0 g • Soluble starch 2.5 g • Agar (Difco) 10.0 g • MOPS buffer 500 ml c. **Liquid phase:** • Trypticase soy broth (Difco) (TSB) 30.0 g • Gelatin (Difco) 10.0 g • MOPS buffer 500.0 ml	**Solid phase** 1. Dissolve agar and starch in the MOPS buffer by heating in a magnetic stirrer – heater placing a magnetic bar in the flask 2. Add charcoal, keep it in suspension by continuous heating. 3. While stirring to keep the charcoal in suspension, dispense 5.0 ml to each 20 ml serum bottle. 4. Cap each bottle with a piece of aluminium foil and autoclave in metal baskets at 121°C for 20 minutes. 5. Remove from the autoclave and slant the baskets until the bottles cool, so that the apex of the agar reaches the shoulder of each bottle. **Liquid phase** 1. Heat the TSB to dissolve the gelatin avoiding coagulation. 2. Autoclave at 121°C for 15 minutes. 3. Dissolve by mixing vigorously in 500 ml or less of MOPS buffer. 4. Pass through a 0.22 μ membrane filter to sterilize.

(Contd.)

(Contd.)

Ingredient	Preparation of the medium
	Complete medium 1. Dispense 5 ml of the broth aseptically into each of the bottles containing the solid-phase slants. 2. Seal with sterile rubber stoppers and aluminium caps.

Proper use of I-I Medium

Before use, check several inoculated bottles for their ability to support meningococcal growth as well as some un-inoculated bottles for sterility at 35°C.

Before inoculation, pre-warm the bottles in the incubator (35°C–37°C) or allow to reach room temperature (25°C–30°C)

Inoculate the T-I medium as follows.

- Remove the aluminium cap of the T-I bottle with forceps, wipe the rubber stopper with a 70% alcohol swab and use a syringe to aseptically inoculate 0.5–1.0 ml of the CSF into the T-I medium for transport and growth of bacteria.
- Incubate T-I medium at 35–37°C with ~5% CO_2 (or in a candle-jar) until transport is possible.

30.7 PROCESSING OF CSF

Materials required

- CSF specimen preferably distributed in three separate fresh, sterile screw capped bottles.
- Biphasic Trans-isolate (T-I) medium (in case of delay in sending the CSF to the laboratory).
- Blood agar plate (BAP).
- Chocolate agar plate (CAP).
- Gram staining reagents.
- Blood culture media for simultaneous blood culture.

30.8 PROCEDURE

	Performance of tests		Remarks
Day 1	**1. Physical examination**. Appearance of the CSF and interpretation are as under		May give a preliminary report
	Appearance	**Interpretation**	
	Clear and colourless	normal	
	Clear and sparkling with against incident light	high protein content	
	Clear yellowish	old hemolysis	
	Clear red	fresh hemolysis	
	Turbid, blood stained	hemorrhage	
	Turbid, white	high cell or protein content	
	Turbid, clot (after overnight incubation)	fibrin clot formation	

(Contd.)

(Contd.)

	Performance of tests	Remarks
	2. Microscopic examination: Use the well mixed sediment for Gram staining, and capsule swelling test, if applicable. Do grams staining on scraping of septic spots on skin in case of suspected meningococcal meningitis. Use dark ground microscopy for detection of *Leptospira*, in case suspected **Centrifuge the CSF:** Use the sediment for microscopic examination and the supernatant for antigen detection test. **Observation on Gram staining** • *N. meningitidis* may occur intracellularly or extracellularly in Polymorphonuclear (PMN) leukocytes and will appear as Gram-negative, coffee-bean shaped diplococci. • *S. pneumoniae* may occur intracellularly or extracellularly and will appear as Gram-positive, lanceolate diplococci, sometimes occurring in short chains. • *H. influenzae* are small, pleomorphic Gram-negative rods or coccobacilli with random arrangements. **3. Culture for bacteria** • **Directly from CSF:** check the approximate volume of CSF. If it is less than 1 ml, directly streak - inoculate 1–5 drops of the specimen on both BAP and CAP. If the volume is more than 1 ml, centrifuge the specimen at 1000X g for 10–15 minutes and process 1 drop of well mixed sediment for culture on BAP and CAP. • **From T-I medium:** draw approximately 100–200 μl with the sterile syringe minimizing the possibility of contaminating the T-I medium. Using a sterile bacteriological loop, cross-streak the inoculum to obtain single, isolated colonies on each of the BAP and CAP. Sterilize the loop prior to each step of plate streaking process Inoculate a back-up broth (e.g. brain-heart infusion broth with proper supplements) with some of the sediment pellet. Incubate the inoculated agar plates and broth for 18–24 hours at 35–37°C with ~5% CO_2 (or in a candle-jar) **4. Antigen detection:** Use the supernatant for antigen detection by latex agglutination test or by rapid diagnostic test (RDT) for detection of antigens of suspected organisms **Latex agglutination test** 1. Heat the CSF supernatant at 100°C for 3 minutes. 2. Shake the latex reagents gently until homogenous. 3. Place one drop of each latex reagent on a disposable card provided in the kit or a ringed glass slide. 4. Add 30–50 μl of the supernatant of the CSF to each latex reagent.	

(Contd.)

	Performance of tests	Remarks
	5. Rotate by hand for 2–10 minutes. If available, mechanical rotation at 100 rpm is recommended. 6. Examine the agglutination reactions under a bright light without magnification. **Reading the latex agglutination results** • Positive reaction: agglutination (or visible clumping) of the latex particles and slight clearing of the suspension occurs within 2–10 minutes. • Negative reaction: the suspension remains homogeneous and slightly milky in appearance. **Rapid diagnostic test (RDT)** procedure for CSF for *N. meningitidis* and *S. pneumonia* 1. Follow manufacturer's instruction on the package 2. Store RDTs dipsticks at 4°C in a moisture proof bag until use. 3. Place the two dipsticks (RDT1 and RDT2) into two separate tubes (3 ml disposable plastic tubes are recommended) of 150–200 μl of CSF or a reference strain suspension in PBS, pH 7.2 4. Record the chromatographic result on each strip after 10–15 minutes at room temperature (25°C) **Result of RDT** • Appearance of red lines on the dipsticks will indicate whether one of the four meningococcal serogroups has been detected in the CSF. • The upper line on the dipstick is the positive control and should always be present. • A negative result consists of a single upper pink control line only.	
Day 2	Examine the plates for growth. Observe the growth characteristics and colony characteristics. • *Streptococcus pneumoniae*—flat, clear colonies with concave centres and zone of alpha hemolysis. There will be zone of inhibition of growth in presence of an optochin disc. • *Haemophilus influenzae*—tiny, water drop, non-hemolytic colonies on BAP and much larger colonies on CAP. • *N. meningitidis*—colonies of *N. meningitidis* are graey and unpigmented on a BAP and appear round, smooth, moist, glistening, and convex, with a clearly defined edge. *N. meningitidis* appear as large, colourless-to-gray, opaque colonies on a CAP. Identify the organisms by putting up biochemical tests. Put up antibiotic sensitivity test.	May give a final report
Day 3 and subsequent days till visible growth is observed	Same as above	Give a final report

30.9 LABORATORY RECORD OF CSF CULTURE

Record the result of CSF culture as under:

Date	Result	In case of positive meningitis		Teacher's signature
		Organism isolated	*Antibiotic sensitivity*	

31

Bacteriological Examination of Water, Milk, Food and Air

31.1 BACTERIOLOGICAL EXAMINATION OF WATER

31.1.1 Aim

To educate the students the importance of bacteriological examination of water for healthy living.

31.1.2 Learning Outcome

Students learn the importance and methods of bacteriological examination of water in order to exclude the possibility of water borne diseases.

31.1.3 Purpose

Bacteriological examination of water is done:

- To ensure safe supply of water.
- To identify water sources that has been contaminated with potential disease producing organisms.
- To ensure absence of fecal contamination in the water.
- To exclude the possibility of water borne diseases.

31.1.4 Sampling of Water (as Recommended by World Health Organization)

Sampling from a tap or pump outlet

1. Check the tap for uniform flow of water.
2. Wipe off the dirt from outside the mouth of the tap.
3. Flame the mouth of the tap using gas burner, lighter or ignited cotton wool soaked in spirit.
4. Open the tap and allow water to flow at medium rate for 1–2 minutes.
5. Open the sterile container (250 ml bottle with glass stopper or with screw cap) and fill it up to 3/4th of its capacity by holding the bottle under the water jet. For chlorinated water, use the bottle with 0.1 ml of 1.8% sodium thiosulphate solution per 100 ml of water sample.
6. Stopper the container and label it.

Sampling from reservoir/pool, etc.

1. Open the sterile bottle under aseptic conditions.
2. Submerge it to a depth of about 20 cm, with the mouth facing slightly upwards to fill the water. If there is a current, the bottle should face the current.
3. Stopper the bottle and label it.

31.1.5 Methods for Water Analysis

Initial detection of fecal contamination by the presence of *Escherichia coli* consists of three steps
1. Presumptive coliform test
2. Confirmatory test for fecal *Escherichia coli* (Eijkman test)
3. Complete test

31.1.5.(a) Presumptive Coliform Test

1. Depending on the quality of water, take 5 samples of water each of 50 ml volume, 10 ml volume and 1 ml volume.
2. Add the water samples to tubes of MacConkey broth containing bromocresol purple indicator and Durham's tube.
3. Incubate at overnight at 37°C and examine the tubes for colour change to yellow and gas production in the Durham's tube.

31.1.5.(b) Confirmatory Test for Fecal *Escherichia coli* (Eijkman Test)

1. Inoculate from each tube showing acid and gas production in the presumptive tests on each of two sets   of lactose broth with an inverted Durham's tube pre heated at 37° C and 44°C and tryptone water medium pre-heated to 44°C.
2. Incubate each set of inoculate lactose medium overnight at 37°C and at 44°C and tryptone water at 44°C in a water bath along with control strains of *Esch. coli* and *Klebsiella aerogenes* for 24 hours.
3. Confirm the presence of *Escherichia coli* by growth at 44°C, colony characteristics and IMViC (indole, methyl red, Voges-Proskauer and citrate utilization) tests.
4. Refer to the table of most probable numbers (MPN).
5. Determine the confirmed coliform count from the combination of positive and negative results for gas production at 37°C read the value of MPN of Coliform bacilli per 100 ml of water.
6. Determine the confirmed *E.coli* count from the combination of positive and negative results for gas and indole production at 44°C read the value of MPN of *E.coli* per 100 ml of water.

31.1.5(c) Complete Test with Bacterial Counting

Medium used for counting is **yeast extract agar**

Composition	Preparation
• Yeast extract 3 g • Peptone 5 g • Agar 15 g Chlorine free distilled water 1litre	1. Dissolve the ingredients in water 2. Adjust the final pH to 7.2 when cooled 3. Dissolve agar-agar by heating 3. Distribute in 10 ml quantities in screw capped bottles. 4. Sterilize by autoclaving at 121°C for 20 minutes

For bacterial counting, take 7 test tubes each with 9 ml of lactose broth
- Make 10 fold serial dilution of water in lactose broth by sequentially transferring 1 ml from the water sample to each tube marked as 1, 2, 3, 4. Transfer 1 ml from tube 1 to tube 2, mix well, transfer 1 ml from tube 2 to tube 3, mix well, transfer 1 ml from tube 3 to tube 4, mix well and transfer 1 ml from tube 4 to tube 5. Discard 1 ml from tube 6. Keep tube 7 as a control without adding any water sample in the lactose broth.

- Dilution in the tube 1 shall be 0.1, in tube 2, it is 0.01, in tube 3, it is 0.001, in tube 4, it is 0.0001 and in tube 5 it is 0.00001 (Fig. 31.1).
- Pour 1 ml from each tube on each of yeast extract agar media and a MacConkey media. Incubate overnight at 37°C.
- Count the number of colonies. Multiply the number of colonies with the dilution used.
- Use statistical tables to derive the most proable no. MPN of organisms in the original sample.

The unit of measurement is cfu/ml (or colony forming units per millilitre) and relates to the original sample. Most probable number (MPN) is the total number of colonies seen per 100 ml of water.

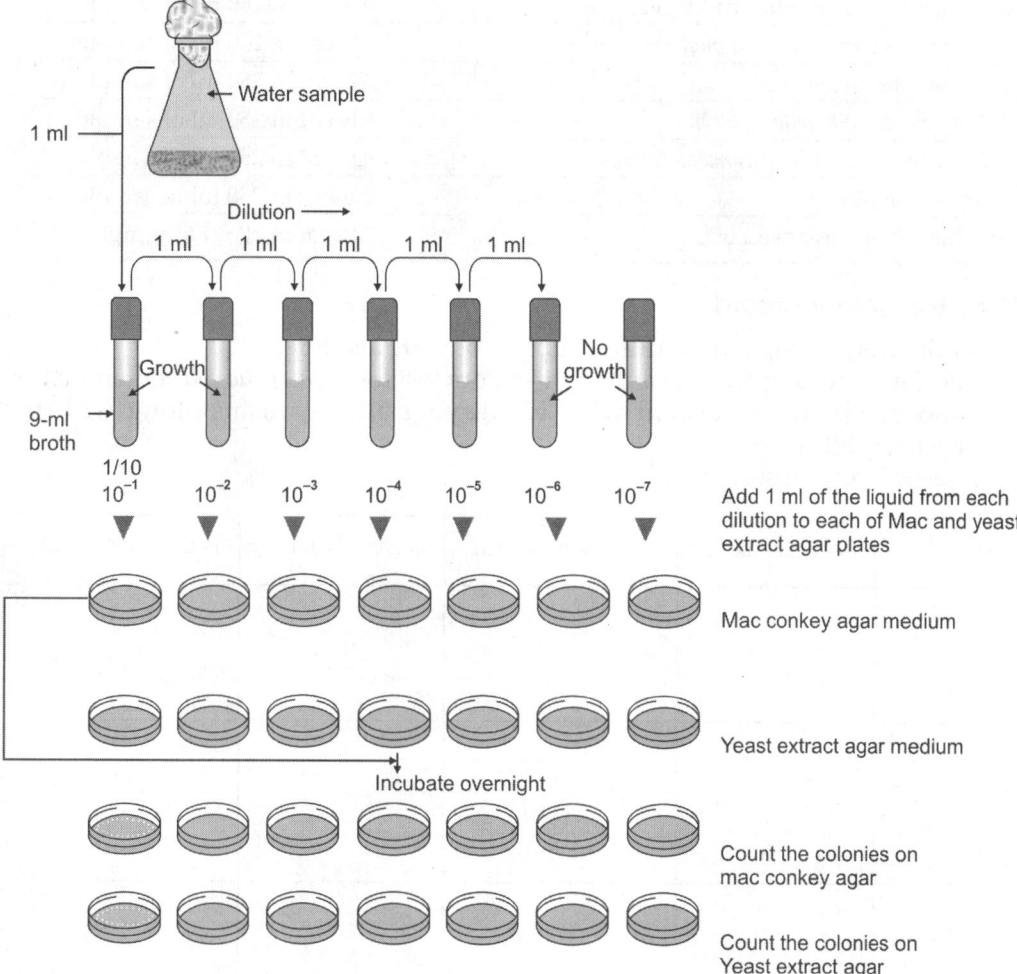

Fig. 31.1: Serial dilution of the water sample and subsequent culture for bacterial counting

Membrane filtration

More recent method is to vacuum filter the serially diluted water samples through membrane filters having a printed millimeter grid printed on it and placing these filters on the nutrient agar plate. Counting may be automated or can be done manually.

31.1.6 Pathogen Analysis

In case the water sample shows contamination with coliform bacteria, depending on requirement, look for specific pathogens like *Salmonella typhi* and *Salmonella typhimurium*. In tropical areas, analysis for *Vibrio cholerae* is also routinely undertaken.

Permissible limit of microbial population in drinking water is given in Table 31.1.

Table 31.1: Permissible limit of microbial population in drinking water	
Organism	*Requirement*
Aerobic bacterial count at 20°C to 22°C, 72 hours incubation	shall not exceed 100/ml
at 37°C, 24 hours incubation	shall not exceed 20/ml
Escherichia coli and other coli form bacteria	Absent in 250 ml of sample
Fecal *Streptococcus* and *Staphylococcus aureus*	Absent in 250 ml of sample
Pseudomonas areuginosa	Absent in 250 ml of sample
Salmonella and *Shigella*	Absent in 250 ml of sample
Vibrio cholerae and *V. parahaemolyticus*	Absent in 250 ml of sample
Yeast and mold	Absent in 250 ml of sample
Sulphite reducing anaerobes	Absent in 50 ml of sample

31.1.7 Laboratory Record

1. Take water sample from different parts of your institute.
2. Perform presumptive test and confirmatory test for *Escherichia coli* contamination and complete the examination identifying all organisms along with the bacteriological counting.
3. Record your observation.

Date	Source of water	Organism isolated	Bacterial count	Teacher's signature

31.2 BACTERIOLOGICAL EXAMINATION OF MILK

31.2.1 Aim

To educate the students the necessity of bacteriological examination of milk for healthy living and the methods for its examination.

31.2.2 Learning Outcome

Students learn to carry out different procedures for checking the milk quality for excluding the possibility of milk borne diseases.

31.2.3 Purpose

Bacteriological examination of milk is done to examine the suitability of milk for consumption.

Pathogenic organism	Normal flora
Escherichia coli, Streptococcus pyogenes, Mycobacterium tuberculosis, Salmonella, Brucella abortus, Campylobacter, Listeria monocytogenes, etc.	Streptococcus lactis, Lactobacillus, Candida albicans (in yoghurt) Bacterial count < 3 × 1000 cfu/ml

31.2.4 Method

Examination of milk consists of following steps:

In Raw Milk

- Microscopic examination of Gram stained smear to see the presence and Gram reaction of bacteria and acid fast stain, smear if tuberculosis is suspected in the cow.
- Qualitative analysis by methylene blue reduction time (MBRT).
- Culture for isolation and identification of *Staphylococcus aureus* and *Salmonella*.
- Quantitative assessment of milk.

In Pasteurized Milk

- Microscopic examination of Gram stained smear to see the presence and Gram reaction of bacteria.
- Culture on agar plate and determination plate count at 21°C.
- Performing tests for coliform, *Listeria*, *Salmonella* and *Staphylococcus*.

Methylene Blue Reduction Time

1. Add 1 ml of methylene blue (1:25000) to 10 ml of the milk sample.
2. Seal the tube and slowly invert the contents three times for proper mixing.
3. Incubate in a water bath at 35°C.
4. Observe the mixture for decolourisation at intervals of 30 minutes

Result (Interpretation may vary)

MBRT	Quality of milk
30 minutes–2 hours	Poor
2–6 hrs	Fair
6–8 hrs	Good
> 8 hrs	Excellent

Culture

For coliform organisms

1. Uniformly spread 0.1 ml of milk on a MacConkey agar plate.
2. Incubate at 37°C.
3. Identify the organisms by colony characteristics and biochemical reactions.

Viable counting

1. **Take Ringer solution** (composition: 7.2 g NaCl, 0.37 g KCl, 0.17 g $CaCl_2$, pH 7.3–7.4 dissolved in one litre of distilled water.)
2. Make 10 fold serial dilution of the milk in Ringer's solution in test tubes from an initial dilution of 1 ml milk added to 9 ml of Ringer solution.
3. Take 1 ml quantity from each dilution, mix with molten and cooled agar medium, shake well and pour plates.
4. Incubate the plates at 37°C for overnight.
5. Count the number of colonies and express the number as number of colony forming unit (cfu) per ml of milk.

31.2.5 Permissible Number of Bacteria

Type of milk	Permissible limit
Pasteurized milk Maximum limit of total count *Staphylococcus aureus,* *Escherichia coli* Listeria	3×1000 cfu/ml of milk < 20 cfu/ml of milk < 10 cfu/ml of milk none in 25 ml of milk
Long shelf life milk	10 cfu/ml of milk

31.2.6 Experiment and Record

1. Obtain milk sample from different sources: Raw milk, pasteurized milk, milk from the kitchen, canteen, etc.
2. Process each sample for determining methylene blue reduction time, culture and bacterial counting.
3. Record your observation in the following table:

Date	Source of milk	Organism isolated	Colony count	Remarks

31.3 BACTERIOLOGICAL EXAMINATION OF FOOD

31.3.1 Aim

To make the students aware of the methods for checking the quality of food and also methods for diagnosis of cases of food poisoning.

31.3.2 Learning Outcome

Students learn to carry out bacteriological examination of different food materials to ensure the quality of food and also to exclude food poisoning.

31.3.3 Purpose

- To check the presence of causative bacterial agent for food poisoning, e.g. *Salmonella* (in poultry, meat and meat products, egg and egg products), *Campylobacter* (in inadequately pasteurized milk), *Clostridium perfringens* (in meat products), *Clostridium botulinum* (in home preserved meat or vegetables), *Bacillus cereus* (in rice and rice products), *Staphylococcus* (in ham, milk products), contamination with *Shigella*, *Escherichia coli*, *Vibrio*, etc.
- To assess whether the food was produced, handled or stored correctly.
- To assess if the food would be a health risk, if consumed.

31.3.4 Procedure

Bacteriological examination of food involves following steps:

- Macroscopic examination of food–look for evidence of fungal growth, check food consistency, odour, etc.

- Sampling of food.
- Homogenization of food.
- Microscopic examination with Gram staining.
- Culture for aerobic colony count.
- Detection of enterotoxin.

Materials required

- Sterile container for food collection.
- Sterile knives, spoons, forceps, spatula.
- Sterile homogenizer.
- Sterile phosphate buffered water for homogenization of food.
- Sterile pipettes of different capacities.
- Sterile blood agar and MacConkey agar plates.

Method

1. Collection of specimen

- Take representative portions of the food with a sterile knife/spoon/forceps/spatula depending on the type of food to be examined.
- Transfer the food material aseptically in a clean, wide mouth, leak-proof, dry and sterile metal container with cap or in a plastic bag (for dry unfrozen materials) that can be sealed.

2. Blending and homogenization: Aseptically weigh approximately 50 g of the sample and blend it in a sterilized blender head with about 450 ml of sterile phosphate buffered water for 2 minutes.

3. Microscopic examination: Make film with the blended food sample. Heat-fix the smear and perform Gram staining.

4. Culture for aerobic colony count (ACC)—ACC is not done for the foods naturally containing high levels of bacteria, e.g. milk products, salami, etc.).

   a. Make dilutions of original homogenate promptly in 10 fold dilutions with sterile phosphate buffered water, using sterile pipettes that deliver required volume accurately.

   b. Shake each dilution vigorously for approximately 30 times, mix with molten agar medium cooled to 50°C and pour plates. Keep the plates at a leveled surface for agar to solidify.

   c. Incubate for 48 hrs at 35°C.

Identify the organism and count the number of colonies for each dilution.

5. Detection of enterotoxin: Demonstrate the enterotoxin production by the isolate by doing agar diffusion using specific antisera against the toxin produced by the organism or by ELISA (Enzyme linked immunosorbent assay) or by PCR (Polymerase chain reaction).

31.3.5 Reporting Results

Results are reported as:

- **Satisfactory: The bacteria found are at acceptable levels;**
- Borderline of acceptability: Levels of bacteria is higher than they expected level.
- Unsatisfactory: This indicates problems with food handling.
- Unacceptable/potentially hazardous: Consumption of this food may cause illness. Immediate action is required. For permissible levels, may refer ICMSF (International Commission on Microbiological Specification for Foods) document.

31.3.6 Experiment and Laboratory Records

1. Take different food samples from the kitchen.
2. Blend them in sterile phosphate buffered saline.
3. Make serial dilution.
4. Culture in appropriate agar medium.
5. Record your observation.

31.4 BACTERIOLOGICAL EXAMINATION OF AIR

31.4.1 Aim

To educate the students the methods for performing bacteriological examination of air in order to control air-borne infections.

Date	Type of food handled	Organisms isolated	Number of organisms per ml of food	Remarks

31.4.2 Learning Outcome

Students learn to perform the bacteriological examination of air for ensuring air quality.

31.4.3 Purpose

To detect presence of airborne bacterial and fungal cells that can cause air borne infections, hospital borne infections, or can contaminate sensitive operations in the laboratory or in pharmaceutical units or Bottom of Form in food factories.

31.4.4 Method

Sample collection and incubation
There are two methods of collection of air samples.

31.4.4.1 Passive Sampling (Settle Plates)

Take sterile petridishes containing non-selective agar media, e.g. Sabouraud's agar medium for mold and nutrient agar or blood agar for bacteria, open the plate for usually 1/2 hour to 1 hour, incubate at appropriate temperature (20°C for 3 days for fungus and 37°C for 24 hours) for bacteria and identify the organisms grown on the settle plates.

31.4.4.2 Active Sampling

Active sampling uses the air samplers that can physically draw a known volume of air over, or through, a particle collection device using a fan or pump.

Two main types of active samplers are:

1. **Impinger** or **slit sampler** in which a known volume of air drawn by a suction pump through a slit into the collection broth contained in a small flask. Subsequently the collection medium is used for viable counting.

2. **Impactor sampler** uses a solid medium as the collection surface, e.g. agar, for particle collection. Air is drawn into the collection surface through a sampling head by a pump or a fan. In sieve sampler, air is accelerated through a perforated plate. On receiving the correct volume of air through the sampling head, the agar plate is removed and incubated directly without further treatment. After incubation, counting the number of visible colonies gives the number of colony forming units in the sampled air.

31.4.4.3 Sampling by Filtration

In sampling by filtration, the air is drawn by a pump or vacuum line through a polycarbonate or cellulose acetate membrane. This filter is then directly transferred onto the surface of an agar medium and incubated. Colonies are counted on the next day. Alternatively, the filter may be placed on a gelatin medium that can be dissolved and analysed by culture or rapid methods like PCR or cytometry.

Table 31.2: Relative advantages and disadvantages of different samplers

Type of sampling	Advantage	Disadvantage
Passive sampling: settle plate	• Inexpensive. • Does not require any special equipment. • Useful for giving qualitative analysis. • Provide early warning on air quality.	• Only the organisms which are settling onto the surface during the time of exposure can grow. • This sampling cannot detect smaller particles floating in air. • This sampling is prone to contamination from non-airborne sources. • Longer exposure time may deteriorate the composition of the agar medium. • Cannot sample specific volume of air.
Active sampling: Impinger sampler	• Quantitative microbial counting possible. • Samples can be analyzed faster by other methods including PCR.	• Impingement in liquids may damage some microbial cells. • Lengthy sampling time may allow some cells to multiply in the liquid medium resulting in wrong estimate.

(Contd.)

Table 31.2: Relative advantages and disadvantages of differents samplers (Contd.)

Type of sampling	Advantage	Disadvantage
Active sampling: Impactor sampler	• Convenient to use. • Risk of contamination and variation can be avoided by using pre-poured standard petridishes. • Can handle higher flow rates and the large sample volumes.	• Agar medium may dry out if allowed to remain in the sampler head too long. • Microbial cells may be damaged during the sampling process and lose viability. • Use of a water-soluble polymer gel instead of agar allows the sample to be analysed by rapid techniques such as PCR or cytometry.
Sampling by membrane filtration	• Filtration methods are accurate and reliable. • Portable filtration samplers designed for the pharmaceutical industry are available. • Identification of organisms and bacterial counting.	• Filtration may cause dehydration stress in the trapped microorganisms.

31.4.5 Experiment and Laboratory Record

1. Place Sabouraud's agar plates for fungus and blood agar plates for bacteria on flat surfaces in various test locations, and remove the lid.
2. Leave the agar exposed for 30 minutes to 1 hour. Monitor the exposure time with a timer.
3. Replace the lid, place the plates in a sterile plastic bag, seal and label clearly.
4. Incubate the plates at 37°C for overnight for bacteria and 25°C for 2 to 4 days for fungus.
5. Identify the organisms on the basis of growth character and biochemical reactions.
6. Record your observations.

Date	Sample location	Organisms isolated	Number of cfu	Teacher's signature

Examination of Stool for Diagnosis of Intestinal Parasitic Infection

32.1 AIM

To educate the students the method of examination of wet film preparation of stool sample prepared directly or after concentration for diagnosis of parasitic infections in the intestine and to identify different intestinal parasites.

32.2 LEARNING OUTCOME

Students learn to make wet film preparations with the stool sample, can process the sample for concentration ova of cyst and can identify different stages of intestinal parasites.

32.3 PURPOSE

Stool examination is a direct method for diagnosis of parasitic infection by demonstrating presence of cyst/trophozoite of protozoa and eggs/larva of helminthes.

32.4 COLLECTION OF STOOL

Ensure that the sample has been collected in leak proof, dry, wide waxed cardboard carton with an overlapping lid or plastic cups with snap-in lid before administration of antibiotics or drugs. Ensure that interfering substances like urine, water or soil is not present in the specimen.

Specimen size: Preferably entire passage in a dry container so that soft or mucoid portion can be examined for staining and more formed portion used for concentration. At least 20–30 gm (size of an walnut) in case of formed stool or 2–3 table spoonful, if loose or watery.

Labelling: Label the sample properly with name, age, gender, date and time of passing the sample. Receive in the laboratory as soon as possible.

32.5 DIRECT EXAMINATION OF STOOL

32.5.1 Macroscopic Examination

Describe the consistency as watery (W), loose (L), soft (S) formed (F). Note the presence or absence of proglottids, whole worm, blood, mucous, and other abnormal materials.

32.5.2 Microscopic Examination

Examine the stool sample under the microscope for the presence or absence of helminthic larvae and/or eggs, trophozoites and/or cyst of protozoa, red blood cells, pus cells, Charcot-Leyden crystals, etc.

Wet film preparation
1. Take preferably a 3" × 2" slide (instead of 3" × 1" slide). Divide in two parts with a marker.

2. Place a drop of physiological saline (0.85% NaCl) on one part and 1% iodine solution on the other part (Fig. 32.1).
3. With an applicator stick or toothpick, pick up very small representative portion of stool, emulsify it in each solution. Cover it with a 22 sqmm cover slip of # 1 thickness. The cover slip must not float on the faecal suspension. Remove excess fluid by pressing lightly between two absorbent towels. Ensure that no air bubble is entrapped. The suspension thickness should be sufficient to just read the newspaper print when the slide is placed on it.
4. Examine the entire coverslipped area under the microscope with 10X objective to see the presence of helminthes ova/larva.
5. Examine the saline suspension for identification of helminthes eggs/larva and trophozoites of protozoa and iodine side for identification cyst of protozoa (Figs 32.3 and 32.4).
6. Confirm your finding with 45X objective.

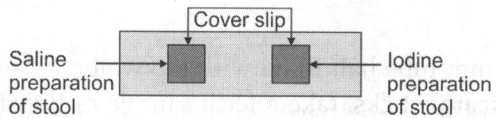

Fig. 32.1: Wet film preparation of stool sample

Collection of sample with National Institute of Health (NIH) swab (Fig. 32.2) for diagnosis of pinworm.

1. Take a rod or tongue depressor or a glass rod and tie a ¾ inch clear cello tape on its one end with the adhesive side of the tape exposed.
2. Press the adhesive surface against several areas of the perianal region a few hours after the person has retired or in the morning before the bowel movement.
3. Keep the sample secured by placing the tied rod or the spatula in another wide mouth tube/container with plug/cap
4. Replace the tape on slide and examine under the microscope.

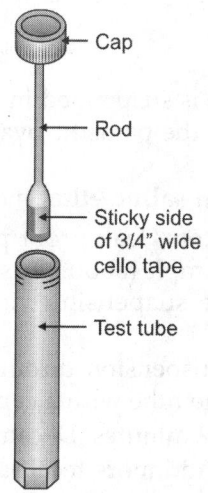

Fig. 32.2: NIH swab

32.6 CONCENTRATION OF STOOL FOR OVA AND CYST

Stool concentration methods are done when the direct wet film preparations show rare or negligible number of parasitic ova or cyst.

Two techniques are used:

1. **Floatation technique**
2. **Sedimentation technique**

32.6.1 Floatation Technique

In this technique, stool sample is suspended in a solution having a specific gravity higher than that of ova or cyst and almost all eggs, larva or cyst float in the solution.

Most common method is the **zinc sulphate floatation technique** in which 330 gm of zinc sulphate is dissolved in 1000 ml of water to give a solution of specific gravity 1.18 or 330 gms of zinc sulphate is dissolved in 700 ml of distilled water to give a resulting specific gravity of 1.20.

Method

1. Take a 100 × 13 mm tube half filled with tap water.
2. Using two applicator sticks, take a fecal sample of the size of a small pea and make a uniform suspension with a small volume of tap water.
3. Add more tap water to make the tube 3/4th full.
4. Centrifuge the suspension at 2500 rpm (650 g) for 1 minute.
5. Pour off the supernatant in a disinfectant container.
6. In case the stool is oily or the supernatant is very cloudy, repeat the washing one more time.
7. Add sufficient zinc sulphate solution to make the tube half full. Make a uniform suspension by re-suspending the sediment in the zinc sulphate solution.
8. Add more zinc sulphate till the tube is filled up to 1 cm from the top.
9. Centrifuge the suspension at 2500 rpm for one minute.
10. Without shaking or spilling, keep the tube in a horizontal rack.

Take the material from the surface film with a wire loop or a capillary pipette and place on a slide for examination. Alternatively, raise the fluid level to form a meniscus on the top and place the coverslip on the meniscus to collect the material for examination under the microscope.

32.6.2 Sedimentation Technique

In this technique, the stool sample is suspended in a solution having specific gravity lower than that of ova an cyst and the parasitic ova, larva and cysts sediments at the bottom.

Most common method **is Formalin-saline-ether** method.

1. Take a beaker or a flat bottom, leak proof paper cup. Make a suspension of approximately 5 gm of the sample (about the size of a groundnut) with sufficient saline so that 10 ml of the suspension yields about 1 ml of sediment on centrifugation.
2. Strain about 10 ml of the suspension through a small funnel containing wet gauge into a 15 ml centrifuge tube with a cap.
3. Centrifuge at 2500 rpm for 2 minutes. Decant supernatant.
4. If the sediment is too little, add more fecal sample and centrifuge after mixing the sample.

5. If the supernatant is very cloudy, wash with the tap water or saline followed by centrifugation two times.
6. To the sediment, add 10% formalin (preferably buffered to a neutral pH) to make the level of the material to 9 ml. Mix the sediment and the buffer thoroughly and allow to stand for 5 minutes.
7. Add 4 ml of ether, stopper the tube and shake vigorously in an inverted position for at least 30 secs. Remove the stopper carefully.
8. Centrifuge at 2000 rpm for two minutes. There will be four layers—namely, ether layer, plug of debris, layer of formalin, sediment (Fig. 32.3)
9. Decant the ether layer and free the plug of debris using a cotton swab.
10. Carefully decant after top three layers into disinfectant solution.
11. With a pipette, mix the remaining sediment with the small amount of fluid draining back from the sides of the tube.
12. Make wet film preparations unstained and stained with iodine.
13. Examine under the microscope.

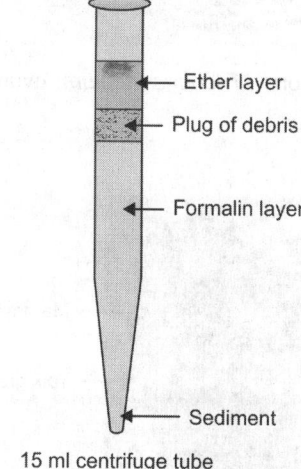

15 ml centrifuge tube

Fig. 32.3: Layers formed in formalin ether saline sedimentation

Morphology of ova and cyst are shown in Figs 32.4 and 32.5.

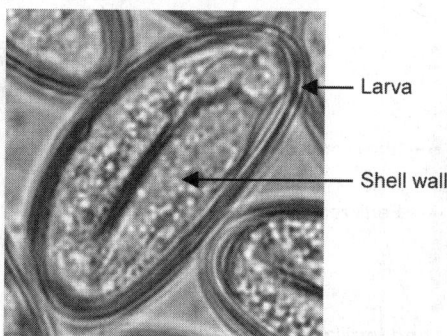

Fig. 32.4: (A) Pinworm (*Enterobius vermicularis*) ovum (*see* colour plate 6)

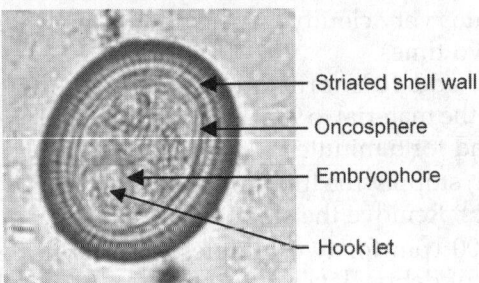

Fig. 32.4: (B) Tapeworm (*Taenia saginata/Taenia solium*) ovum (*see* colour plate 6)

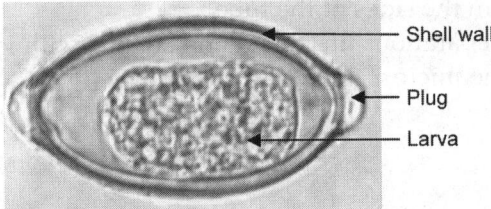

Fig. 32.4: (C) Whipworm (*Trichuris trichiura*) ovum (*see* colour plate 6)

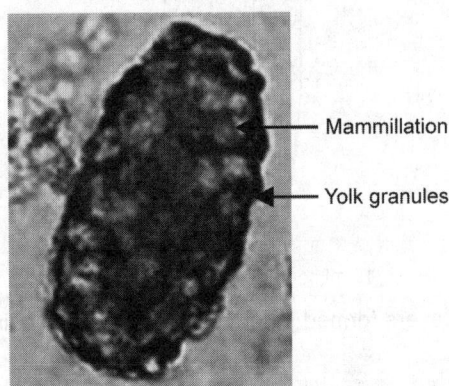

Fig. 32.4: (D) (i) Unfertilized roundworm (*Ascaris lumbricoides*) ovum (*see* colour plate 6)

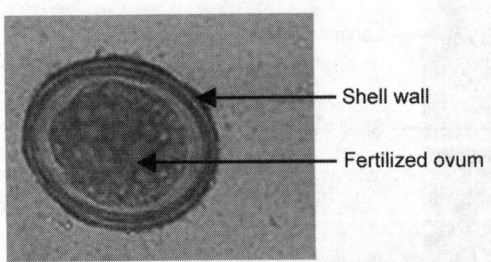

Fig. 32.4: (D) (ii) Decorticated and fertilized ovum of roundworm (*see* colour plate 6)

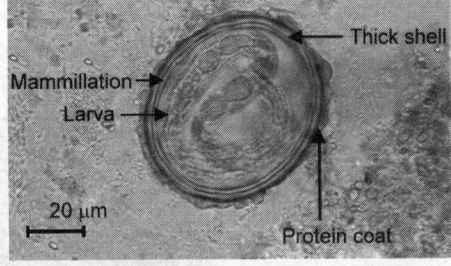

Fig. 32.4: (D) (iii) Embryonated roundworm ovum (*see* colour plate 7)

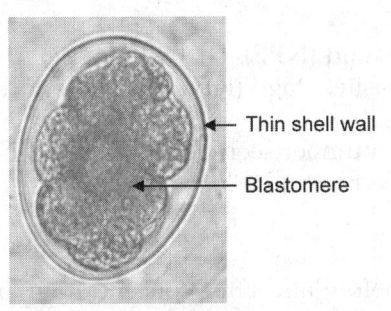

Fig. 32.4: (E) Hookworm (*Ancylostoma duodenale*) ovum (*see* colour plate 7)

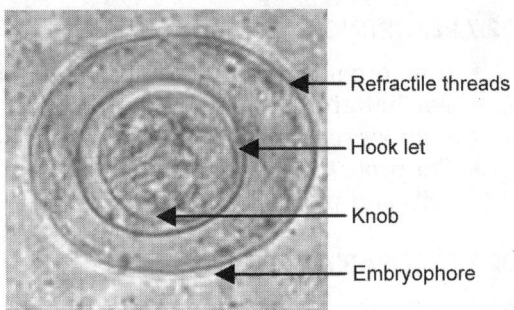

Fig. 3.24: (F) Dwarf tapeworm (*Hymenolepis nana*) ovum (*see* colour plate 7)

Figs 32.4 A to F: Identification of eggs of helminthes in fecal specimen

Entamoeba histolytica (Trophozoite, immature cyst and mature cyst)

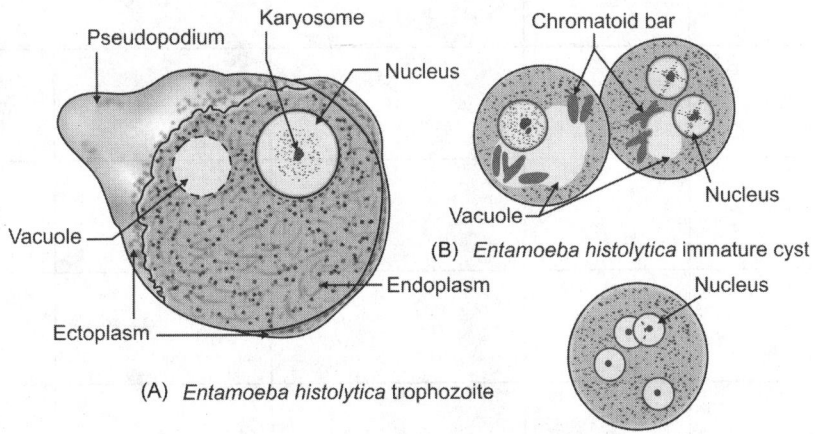

(A) *Entamoeba histolytica* trophozoite

(B) *Entamoeba histolytica* immature cyst

(C) *Entamoeba histolytica* mature cyst

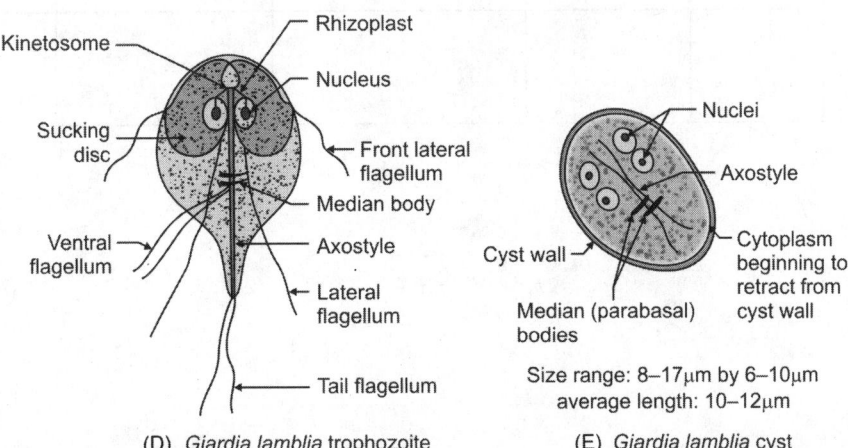

(D) *Giardia lamblia* trophozoite

(E) *Giardia lamblia* cyst

Size range: 8–17μm by 6–10μm
average length: 10–12μm

Fig. 32.5 A to E: Identification of trophozoites and cysts in fecal specimen (A) Trophozoite of *Entamoeba histolytica,* (B and C) Immature and mature cyst of *Entamoeba histolytica,* (D) Trophozoite of Giardia, (E) Cyst of *Giardia,*

32.7 REPORTING

- If no organism found: Report as no parasite found (NPF).
- **For helminthes**: Report the name of the parasite, stage (larva or egg) and the number seen in the entire cover slipped areas.
- **For protozoa**: Report the name, stage and the number seen per HPF. Red blood cells and pus cells, if present, report the number seen/HPF.

32.8 LABORATORY RECORD

Make wet film preparations from stool samples before and after concentration and record your observations.

Date	Method used			Observation and report	Teacher's signature
	Direct	Concentration			
		Floatation	Sedimentation		

33

Laboratory Diagnosis of Fungal Infection

33.1 AIM

To create awareness amongst the students about common fungal contaminations in the laboratory, methods used for microscopic examination of fungus, culture of fungus and the general methods used for laboratory diagnosis of fungal infection.

33.2 LEARNING OUTCOME

Students learn to examine the fungus under the microscopes, can identify the common fungi from their mycelial characteristics, can prepare the culture medium for fungus, understand the importance of the laboratory diagnosis for fungal infection and can carry out the procedure of laboratory diagnosis.

33.3 PURPOSE

- To identify fungi present in the environment as contaminants.
- To confirm superficial fungal infection involving the hair, scalp, palms of the hands, soles of the feet and also of systemic infections.
- To isolate and identify the species of fungus from the specimens.
- To carry out epidemiological studies.

33.4 OBSERVATION OF CHARACTERISTICS OF COMMON FUNGAL CONTAMINATION IN THE LABORATORY

Fungal contaminations in the laboratory arise out of presence of fungi in air, soil, dust, plant debris, etc. Spores get easily transported by air as they are very light.

Fungal contaminants are identified by their mycelial characteristics and by the colour, shape and size of the spores.

Characteristics of common fungi isolated as contaminants in the laboratory are given in Table 33.1.

Table 33.1: Characteristics of common fungi isolated as contaminants in the lab		
Fungus genus	*Presence in the environment*	*Morphological characteristics*
Alternaria	Comes from decaying plant materials. Spores of *Alternaria*	Dark brown spores borne in simple or branched chain. Conidiophore dark and divided by

(Contd.)

Table 33.1: Characteristics of common fungi isolated as contaminants in the lab *(Contd.)*

Fungus genus	Presence in the environment	Morphological characteristics
	species are dispersed by air currents and are usually abundant in outdoor air.	transverse and vertical walls. New spores produced at the tip of previous spore.
Aspergillus	Are abundant in soil, house dust, plant debris	Conidiophores arise from well defined foot cell and terminates by a swollen vesicle bearing flask shaped phialide. Spores are of different colours depending on the species and are produced in long chains from phialides.
Fusarium	Abundantly found in soil and living and dead plants	Spores (conidia)are colourless and are canoe shaped when viewed laterally. Foot cell is distinct and divided by several cross walls. Conidiophores are often clustered. Phialides tapered. Microconidium attached on canoe shaped structure.
Mucor	Common almost everywhere fungi occur.	Spores (sporangiospores) are large and dark. Sporangiophores are upright with the columella holding the sporangia at the tip. Sometimes large,dark

(Contd.)

Table 33.1: Characteristics of common fungi isolated as contaminants in the lab (*Contd.*)

Fungus genus	Presence in the environment	Morphological characteristics
		spores (zygospores) may be produced.
Penicillium	Usually is most abundant genus of fungi in soils. May occur in food producing toxin	Green conidia. Conidiophores are simple or branched and are terminated by flask shaped phialides. The spores (conidia) are produced in dry chains from the tips of the phialides, with the youngest spore at the base of the chain, and are nearly always green. Branching is an important feature for identifying *Penicillium* species. (painting brush type) a. One stage branch b. Second stage branch c. Three stage branch
Rhizopus	Present almost everywhere with rapidly dispersing spores. Common on decaying fruits, soil, and house dust.	Sporangia is dark containing dark to pale spores. Columella on sporangiophore is large. At the base of sporangiophore are the root like rhizoids. Often spreading by means of aerial, creeping stolons

33.5 PREPARATION OF VARIOUS CULTURE MEDIA USED IN MYCOLOGY

33.5.1 Sabouraud's Agar Medium for Primary Isolation of Fungus from Clinical Materials

Preparation

Ingredient	Method of preparation
• Peptone 10 g • Glucose 40 g • Distilled water 1 litre • Agar-agar 20 g pH 5.4	1. Weigh the ingredients. 2. Dissolve the ingredients in water by gentle heating. 3. Make up the volume of the medium to 1 litre. 4. Adjust the pH to 5.4. 5. Add agar-agar. Dissolve the agar by free steaming or by continuous stirring by placing the container in a water bath.

(*Contd.*)

(Contd.)

Ingredient	Method of preparation
	6. Filter through layers of gauge piece.
	7. Distribute in bottles.
	8. Sterilize by autoclaving at 8 lbs pressure for 30 minutes.
	9. Cool a part of sterile molten media at an approximate temperature of 52°C. Keep remaining media in bottles.
	10. Distribute part of cooled sterile medium in sterile petridishes with sterile precautions.
	11. Store at 4°C.
	Depending on specific requirements, antibiotics may be added to the media to suppress bacterial growth.

33.5.2 Sodium Pyruvate Agar Medium for Cultivation of *Nocardia*

Composition	Preparation
• Sodium pyruvate 2.5 g • Yeast extract 0.25 g • Indicator bromocresol purple (1.6 g bromocresol purple solution dissolved in 100 ml of 95% ethyl alcohol 0.50 ml) • Distilled water 500 ml • Agar 10 g pH 6.8	1. Dissolve the ingredients in 500 ml of water by gentle heating, if required. 2. Adjust the pH to 6.8. 3. Add agar. Dissolve by steaming. 4. Sterilize the media in the autoclave at 121°C for 15 mins. 5. Cool. 6. Pour plates.

Quality Control

- Check the sterility of the prepared agar medium by keeping one plate in the incubator for overnight. There should not be any growth after incubation.
- Check the ingredients by inoculating one plate with known fungus/*Nocardia*. There should be good growth.

33.6 EXPERIMENT AND LABORATORY RECORDS

1. Take several plates of Sabouraud's agar media.
2. Keep them open at various places of the laboratory for five minutes.
3. Close the plates and incubate at 35–37°C overnight.
4. Examine the growth and identify the fungal contaminant.
5. Record your observations.

Date	Location of the sampling plate	Observation after incubation/organism grown	Teacher's signature

33.7 LABORATORY DIAGNOSIS OF FUNGAL INFECTION

Fungal infections are generally of two types (Fig. 33.1)

1. Superficial, cutaneous and subcutaneous infection, i.e. infection of skin, nail, hair, etc.
2. Deep mycoses: These infections are generally seen in patients with diabetes, AIDS, immune suppressed patients viz., after cancer therapy, transplantation, major surgery, etc. The infection may spread in brain, lungs, heart, liver, spleen, kidney.

33.7.1 Sample Collection

General Rules for Sample Collection

- Collect specimen before starting any antifungal treatment.
- Collect specimen as early as possible from the onset of the symptoms.
- Collect morning sample, whenever applicable.
- With larger quantity of specimen, yield always increases.

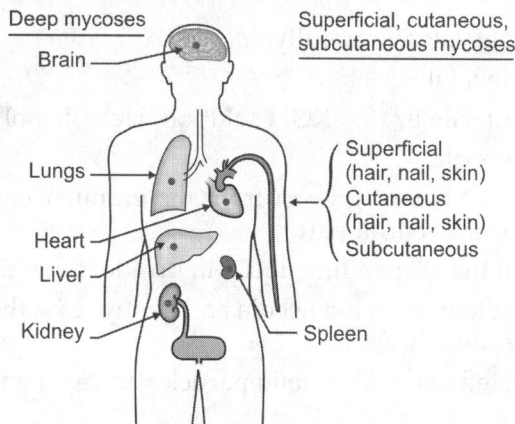

Fig. 33.1: Location of fungal infections

Sample Collection for Superficial Infections

Skin scraping

- With an alcohol wipe, remove any trace of skin cosmetics or medication.
- Examine the area carefully. In case of multiple lesions, choose the most recent one for scraping.
- Scrape the skin using a sterile scalpel.
- Place in the sample in the specimen container.

Nail Cuttings/Scrapings

- Clean the nail with an alcohol wipe.
- Choose the white degenerating portion beneath the nail for collection of the sample.
- Scrape the crumbling debris under the nail plate with the blunt end of a sterile lancet.
- Put the scrapings in the laboratory specimen container.
- Collect nail clippings also.

Hair Specimens
- Carefully observe the affected area of the scalp with a light source.
- Use tweezers to pluck hairs from the affected area.
- Scrape the affected area using a sterile scalpel.
- Put the scrapings in the laboratory specimen container.

Subcutaneous lesions
- **Abscess:** Aspirate the sample with sterile needle and syringe and place in the specimen container.
- **Open wound:** Collect the material with sterile swab.

Deep Mycoses

Collect the specimen depending on the location of infection, viz., urine, blood, CSF, pleural fluid, synovial fluid, bronchial aspirate, tissue, etc.

33.7.2 Examination of Wet Film Preparation

Tease Preparation

1. Examine the fungal colony carefully.
2. Take a slide and label it.
3. Place two drops of saline/10% KOH solution/lactophenol cotton blue.
4. Sterilize loop or needle.
5. Cut a small piece of fungal growth from the granular or coloured part of the colony away from the central part.
6. Place the piece on the suspending liquid in upside down position.
7. Hold the fungal colony with the needle and gently tease the inverted side of the sample in the suspending fluid.
8. After enough teasing, remove all solid particles and agar and discard them in the disinfectant.

33.7.3 STAINING TECHNIQUES FOR DIRECT DEMONSTRATION OF FUNGAL PREPARATION

Preparation of solution
a. 10% potassium hydroxide (used for examining the wet film preparation)

Composition	Preparation
• Potassium hydroxide 10 g (digests tissue cells and clarify it) • Glycerol 20 ml (prolongs shelf life of the reagent, prevents crystallization) • Distilled water 80 ml	Dissolve potassium hydroxide in water, add glycerol, filter, sterilize, store in a sterile container.

b. Lactophenol cotton blue used for staining

Composition	Preparation
• Lactic acid 20 ml (cleaning agent • Phenol crystals 20 g (disinfectant) • Cotton blue 0.05 g • Glycerol 40 ml (prevent drying)	Dissolve the ingredients (except cotton blue) by gentle heating. Add cotton blue.

Examination of the Stained Preparations

- Lactophenol cotton blue slide: Cover the teased material gently with a cover slip, heat briefly to stain the cell wall of the fungi and examine under 10× objective.
- India ink preparation: Add a drop of India ink on the wet film preparation of the fungal material, cover with a cover slip (22 × 40 mm) and press gently, allow to stand for a few minutes and examine under 10X objective.

33.7.4 Processing of the Specimen

	Performance of tests	*Remarks*
Day 1	Examine the specimen under the microscope with lactophenol cotton blue and India ink for preliminary identification. Inoculate on appropriate medium (SDA, BAP, CAP, BHIA) and incubate. Send part of the tissue for histopathological examination.	Give preliminary report based on microscopic examination.
Day 2 and subsequent days till growth occurs	Examine the growth. Identify the specific fungi by antigen antibody reaction (latex agglutination test), production of specific metabolite, capsule swelling test, presence of cell wall marker, e.g., beta-1,3, glycan, enolase, DNA detection by PCR technology, etc. Put up antifungal susceptibility test.	
Next day	Identify the isolate.	Give final report

33.8 LABORATORY RECORD

Take specimens from various sites of the body. Isolate and identify the fungus. Record your findings:

Date	Specimen used	Organism isolated	Teacher's signature

34

Antigen–Antibody Reactions

34.1 AIM

To familiarize the students about various antigen–antibody reactions used in the diagnosis of microbial infections.

34.2 LEARNING OUTCOME

The students can carry out different diagnostic procedures based on antigen-antibody reactions.

34.3 DIAGNOSTIC TESTS

34.3.1 Antistreptolysin O Titre (ASOT)

Purpose

Antistreptolysin O titre (ASOT) is used to assist in the diagnosis of scarlet fever, rheumatic fever, and glomerulonephritis caused by β-hemolytic streptococci.

Principle

Streptolysin O is an immunogenic, oxygen-labile hemolytic toxin produced by most strains of group A and many strains of groups C and G streptococci. Main function of streptolysin O is to cause β-hemolysis. Anti-streptolysin O (ASO or ASLO) is the antibody produced in the body against streptolysin O. In ASOT, inhibition of hemolysis by patient's serum when added to a mixture of rabbit or human blood and commercial streptolysin O is assessed.

Materials Required

- Patient's blood collected in 3.8% sodium citrate dehydrate (1 volume blood to 1.2 volume citrate).
- Streptolysin O reagent in 10 ml vial.
- Fresh rabbit blood or human erythrocytes (O negative).
- Phosphate buffered saline (pH 6.5–6.7).
- Internal control serum (one with high titre and one with low titre) obtained from a reference library.
- Microtitre plates
- Incubator
- Timing device

Method

1. Prepare a 1:10 dilution of patient's serum by adding 50 μl of serum to 450 μl of phosphate buffered saline. Cover the tubes and inactivate at 56°C for 30 minutes
2. In microtitre plates, add 50 μl of PBS in each well of three raws.
3. Make serial dilution starting with 50 μl of patient's sera in one row of the microtitre plate. In other two rows, make serial dilutions of positive control sera having high titre and negative control serum having low titre.
4. Add 25 μl of SO reagent to each plate. Incubate at 37°C for 30 minutes.
5. Add 25 μl of erythrocyte suspension to all wells. Re-incubate at 37°C for 45 minutes.
6. Examine the wells for hemolysis.

Result: ASO titre is the inverse of the highest serum dilution that inhibits the action of streptolysin O. This is the serum dilution of the last well showing no hemolysis.

A raised or rising levels of ASO indicates past or present infection. Normal ranges (Generally, an ASO test value below 200 is considered normal. In preschool-aged children, the test value should be less than 100) may vary from laboratory to laboratory and by age. False positives can result from liver disease and tuberculosis.

34.3.2 Test for C Reactive Protein

C reactive protein is named because of its ability to react with somatic C polysaccharide of *Streptococcus pneumoniae*. It is produced in the liver. The level of CRP rises whenever there is an inflammation in the body

Purpose

C reactive protein test is a non-specific test used for detection or monitoring tissue injury or infection somewhere in the body. Changes in the serum level of CRP with time from the same patient can be used as an index of recovery.

Principle

CRP test is based on the latex-agglutination method involving the immunological reaction between CRP as an antigen and the corresponding antibody coated on the surface of biologically inert latex particles.

Reagents and Materials Required

- CRP latex reagent: Polystyrene latex particles coated with anti-human CRP and suspended in buffer and 0.1% sodium azide preservative. Shake well prior to use.
- CRP positive control: Human serum that contains CRP and 0.1% sodium azide as preservative.
- CRP negative control: Human serum without CRP that contains 0.1% sodium azide as preservative.
- Glycine buffer concentrate (20×): To be diluted 1 part with 19 parts distilled water.
- Disposable pipettes.
- Glass test slide.
- Serological pipettes.
- Test tubes 12 × 75 mm.
- Timer.
- Distilled water.

Specimen Collection

Use only fresh patient serum as the specimen. In case there is a delay in carrying out the test after collecting blood, keep the serum refrigerated. If testing is to be prolonged in excess of 24 hours, keep the serum in the freezer as bacterial contamination may cause protein denaturation.

Test Procedure

Method I (Qualitative method)

1. Bring all reagents, controls and serum samples to room temperature.
2. Shake the CRP latex reagent gently before use. Deliver one drop of reagent to the test circle. Using the disposable pipettes, add one drop of the undiluted patient serum onto the same circle and mix both together.
3. Run positive and negative controls with each series of test sera in the same way as in step 2.
4. Rotate slide back and forth for 2 minutes and read result under an indirect oblique light source.

Method II (Semi-quantitative method)

1. Set up at least 5 test tubes and label 1:2, 1:4, 1:8, 1:16, 1:32, and 1:64, etc.
2. Use diluted glycine-saline buffer to serially dilute patient's serum.
3. Repeat all steps as in qualitative method using these new samples.

Results: Positive reaction is indicated by agglutination. Repeat negative results using a diluted serum sample in case prozone effect is suspected due to antigen excess. For the semi-quantitative method, multiplication of the dilution factor with 6 mg/litre will yield the approximate level of CRP in the serum sample.

Dilution	Concentration of CRP (mg/litre)
1:1	6
1:2	12
1:4	24
1:8	48

Limitation

- Weak reactions may occur with slightly elevated or markedly elevated CRP concentrations.
- A prozone phenomena (antigen excess) may cause false negatives reaction. It is advisable, to check all negative sera by retesting at a 1:10 dilution.
- Reaction times longer than specified period may produce false positive reactions due to a drying effect.
- Strongly lipemic or contaminated sera can cause false positive reactions.
- Only serum should be used in this test.

Expected Values

Normal adult levels of CRP are less than 12 mg/L. Trace levels of CRP had been reported in the sera of apparently healthy adults and normal children.

The CRP level can increase significantly (> 10 fold) above the normal values with the onset of a substantial inflammatory stimulus.

34.3.3 Rheumatoid Factor

Purpose: Rheumatoid factor (RF) test detects diseases like rheumatoid arthritis, hepatitis, tuberculosis, infections mononucleosis, syphilis, malaria, cirrhosis and chronic active hepatitis and autoimmune diseases, e.g. systemic lupus erythematosus (SLE),

Principle

Rheumatoid factors are antibodies directed against Fc portion of human IgG. A rheumatoid factor (RF) blood test measures the amount of the RF antibody present in the blood.

Procedure

RF titre can be determined by latex agglutination test, nephelometry, solid phase radioimmunoassay or enzyme linked immunosorbent assay (ELISA).

Latex Agglutination Test

Materials Required

- Patient's serum (only fresh serum or serum stored at + 2°C to + 8°C for no longer than 72 hours).
- Polystyrene latex particles coated with heat inactivated IgG (commercially available).
- Borate buffer, pH 8.2.
- Incubator
- Pipette
- Timer

Preparation of borate buffer: Solution A: 0.2 M solution of boric acid (dissolve 12.4 g of boric acid in 1000 ml of distilled water).

Solution B: 0.05 M solution of borax (dissolve 19.05 g of borax (also known as sodium borate) in 1000 ml of distilled water).

50 ml of solution A + 7.3 ml of solution B gives a pH of 8.2

Procedure

1. Make a master dilution of patient's serum by adding 0.5 ml serum to 1 ml of borate buffer.
2. Take 8 tubes. Add 1 ml of borate buffer to each tube.
3. Make a serial two fold dilutions in borate buffer by transferring 0.5 ml of the master dilution of patient's serum to the first tube, transferring 0.5 ml from the first tube to second tube and so on. Discard 0.5 ml from the 7th tube. Do not add any diluted serum in the 8th tube. This serves as a control.
4. Add 1 ml of latex particles coated with heat inactivated IgG to each tube. Incubate at 56°C for 2 hours in the water bath. Observe for agglutination. Record the maximum dilution till which agglutination is seen. This is the RF titer.

Nephelometry measures the degree of blocking of light by the serum sample in the tube. A high level of RF causes the sample to be cloudy, so less light passes through the tube than when the RF level is low.

Radioimmunoassay: In this method, patient's serum is coated in polystyrene tubes. They are incubated with human IgG. After repeated washing, antihuman antibody tagged with radioactive iodine, I^{125} is added and incubated. After washing, the tubes are read through gamma counter for getting the value of count per minute.

ELISA: Method is similar to that of RIA. Instead of radioisotope, enzyme tagged antibody is used. The result is seen by measuring the colour of the product of enzyme reaction.

The results of the rheumatoid factor (RF) test may be reported in titers or units:

Normal value of RF

Titers Less than 1:80

Units Less than 60 units per milliliter (U/mL).

34.3.4 Venereal Disease Research Laboratory Test

Purpose

Venereal disease research laboratory (VDRL) test is a screening test for presumptive laboratory diagnosis of syphilis. Diagnosis is further confirmed by demonstrating the presence of *T.pallidum* under dark field microscopy or by confirmatory tests like *Treponema pallidum* immobilization (TPI) test.

Principle

VDRL test is a slide flocculation test which detects non-treponemal (reagin) antibodies in the serum. With minor modifications it can be done on cerebrospinal fluid also.

Materials Required

VDRL test on patient's serum

- Patient's serum: Heat the serum at 56°C for 30 minutes immediately before the test. If there is a gap of 4 hours after heating, reheat the serum at 56°C for 10 minutes (inactivation)
- Antigen: The antigen is an alcoholic solution containing 0.03% cardiolipin, 0.9% cholesterol and purified lecithin. Buffered saline is also supplied alongwith the commercial preparation for preparing antigen suspension.
- Antigen delivery needle: 18 or 19 gauge needle, with cut tips (without bevel) or 23 gauge with bevel attached to a 1 ml syringe to ensure that 60 drops are obtained from 1 ml of antigen suspension.
- VDRL slides.
- Incubator.
- Timer.
- Pipettes.
- Screw capped bottle.
- VDRL slide shaker

Procedure

Preparation of working suspension of the antigen:

1. Pipette 0.4 ml of buffered saline solution to the bottom of a 30 ml ground glass or screw cap stoppered bottle.
2. Add 0.5 ml antigen directly onto the saline solution within 6 seconds while gently and continuously rotating the bottle on a flat surface.
3. Blow last drop of antigen from pipette without touching pipette to saline solution.
4. Continue rotating bottle for 10 more seconds.
5. Add 4.1 ml buffered saline solution.
6. Place cap on bottle and shake vigorously for approximately 10 seconds and leave it in a dark place for half an hour.
7. The antigen suspension thus prepared should be used within one day.

Test each antigen preparation with known positive and negative serum controls. The antigen particles appear as short rod forms at magnification of about 100×. Aggregation of these particles into large or small clumps is interpreted as degrees of positivity.

Qualitative Serum Slide Test

1. Pipette 0.05 ml of each heated serum into a ring on VDRL glass slide.
2. Set up pre-tested control sera as controls and guide for reading.
3. Add one drop (0.016 ml) antigen suspension to each ring of the VDRL slide.
4. Rotate slides for 4 minutes. Rotation can be on a VDRL shaker or manually. If done manually, the movement should roughly circumscribe a two inch diameter circle 120 times per minute.
5. Read test carefully after rotation and record.

Recording Results

- No clumping or slight clumping: Non-reactive.
- Small clumps: Weakly reactive.
- Medium and large clumps: Reactive.
- Report results of qualitative test only as reactive (R), weakly reactive (WR) or non-reactive (NR).

Quantitative Serum Slide Test

Serum dilutions

1. Pipette 0.5 ml of freshly prepared physiological saline into each of five or more test tubes.
2. Add 0.5 ml of heated serum to tube No. 1, mix well and transfer 0.5 ml to tube No. 2.
3. Continue mixing and transferring until the last tube. Discard 0.5 ml from last tube containing 1 ml.
4. It would give two fold serial dilutions of 1:2, 1:4, 1:8 and so on.
5. Test each serum dilution as described under qualitative serum test.

Reading and recording

- Read test microscopically at 10× as described under qualitative procedure.
- Record the titre as the reciprocal of the last serial dilution that produces a reactive reaction.
- Record the titre as reactive and add the titre in dilutions, e.g. VDRL reactive, 16 dilution.

b. VDRL test on patient's CSF

1. Sensitize the antigen by mixing and gently rotating it with equal amount of 10% sodium chloride solution.
2. Select the needle in such a way that 1 ml gives 100 drops.
3. After mixing with 0.05 ml of CSF, rotate the slides for 8 minutes.

Reporting and recording is similar to that for serum samples.

Presently **rapid plasma reagin (RPR) test** is widely recommended for use in field studies. The test can be carried out on unheated serum or plasma and read with naked eyes. The reagents are commercially available and are economical.

Biological false positives reactions in VDRL may be observed in conditions such as systemic lupus erythematosus, malaria, lepromatous leprosy, infectious mononucleosis, hepatitis, rheumatoid arthritis, collagen disorders, etc.

34.3.5 Widal Test

Purpose

Widal test is done for diagnosis of typhoid and paratyphoid.

Principle

Widal test demonstrates presence of antibodies in patient's serum against various antigen components of cells, [i.e., somatic antigen, (O-antigen) and flagellar antigens (H-antigen)] of *Salmonella typhi* and *Salmonella paratyphi* (Fig. 34.1).

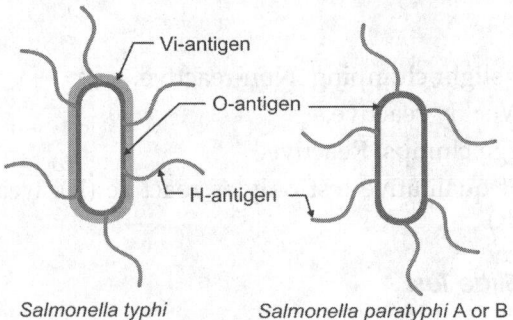

Fig. 34.1: Position of O- and H-antigens in *Salmonella typhi* and *Salmonella paratyphi*

Widal Tube Agglutination Test

Materials Required

- Patient's serum.
- Perfectly clean and dry test tubes.
- Physiological saline.
- Standardized suspension of *Salmonella typhi* O-antigen (To), *Salmonella typhi* flagellar antigen (T_H), *Salmonella paratyphi* flagellar antigen (A_H) and *Salmonella paratyphi* B flagellar antigen (B_H)

Procedure

1. Take 28–32 test tubes.
2. Place them in four different rows.
3. Mark the rows as To, T_H, A_H and B_H.
4. Make a master dilution of 1:10 by adding 0.1 ml serum to 0.9 ml of saline (1:10 dilution).
5. Transfer 0.5 ml of the 1:10 diluted serum from master dilution to the 1st tube of each row, then from the first tube to the second tube, then from second tube to third tube and continue with transferring till the last tube. Discard 0.5 ml of the diluted serum from the last tube of each row.
6. Resultant dilutions shall be 1:20, 1:40, 1:80, 1:160, 1:320, 1:640, etc. (Fig. 34.2)
7. In each row, keep one tube with only 0.5 ml saline as a control tube.
8. Shake the antigen suspensions. Add 0.5 ml of the To antigen in each tube of the first row including the control tube without serum. Add 0.5 ml of T_H antigen in

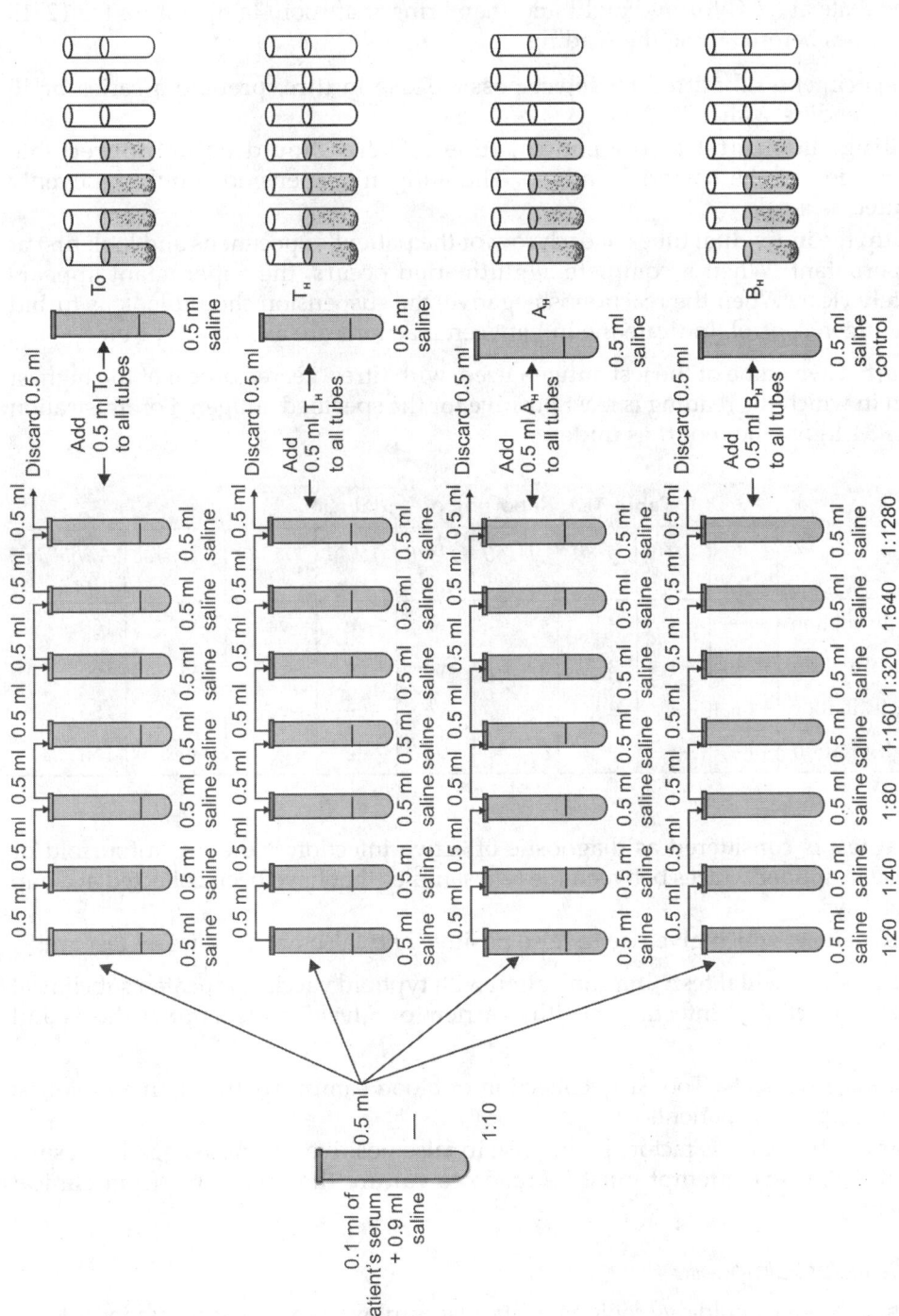

Fig. 34.2: Serial dilution and reading of Widal test

each tube of the second row including the control tube. Add 0.5 ml of A_H antigen in each tube of third row including the control tube and 0.5 ml of B_H antigen in each tube of fourth row including the control tube.
9. Incubate at 37°C for overnight and then bring it at room temperature for 12–15 minutes before taking the reading.

For specimens submitted to detect possible rise in titre, prepare a series of 10 dilutions, ending with 1:5120.

Reading: Look first at the control tubes. There should be no appreciable sedimentation of the bacterial antigen. The antigen suspension should be evenly distributed as a rule.

Pick up the individual tubes of each row of the patient's specimens and look first at the supernatant. When a complete agglutination occurs, the supernatant appears absolutely clear. When the reaction is negative, the suspension should look as turbid as the antigen control. Indicate the in-between reactions are as +, ++. +++ etc.

Report: Give name of the test antigen used, with titres, i.e. reciprocal of the highest dilution in which the reading is least positive for the specified antigen. For illustration at Table 34.1 give the report as under:

Table 34.1: Reporting of Widal test

Dilution	1/20	1/40	1/80	1/160	1/320	1/640	1/1280	Control	Antibody titre
To agglutination	+++	++	+	+	–ve	–ve	–ve	–ve	160
T_H agglutination	+++	++	+	+	–ve	–ve	–ve	–ve	160
A_H agglutination	+++	++	+	+	–ve	–ve	–ve	–ve	160
B_H agglutination	+++	++	+	+	–ve	–ve	–ve	–ve	160

Widal test is considered as diagnostic of active infection if there is a fourfold or more rise in antibody titres between the two samples that have been collected at a gap of 10–14 days.

The situations which give rise to false positive and false negative widal test are:

False positive widal test: Immunization with typhoid vaccine, repeated subclinical infection, past clinical infection, healthy carriers of *S.typhi*, patients of cirrhosis and hepatitis.

False negative tests: Too early collection of blood sample, patients on antibiotics, immune-suppressed patients.

In view of the various factors giving rise to false positive and false negative results in widal test, every attempt must be made to culture the organisms from clinical specimens.

Rapid Tests for Salmonella

a. Using colloidal gold dye conjugate: The test employs a combination of monoclonal antibody/colloidal gold dye conjugate and a polyclonal antibody immobilized on the solid phase. This will selectively identify the *S. typhi* and *paratyphi* A-antigens associated *Salmonella typhi* (typhoid) and *Salmonella paratyphi* (paratyphoid) infections with a high degree of sensitivity and specificity.

b. Using one step *Salmonella typhi/Salmonella paratyphi* test strip pre-coated with anti-Salmonella antibodies on the test line region of the strip for detection of *Salmonella typhi* and *Salmonella paratyphi* in stool/serum/plasma. During testing, the stool/serum/plasma specimen migrates upward on the membrane chromatographically by capillary action to react with anti-Salmonella antibodies on the membrane and generate a coloured line. The presence of this coloured line in the test region indicates a positive result, while its absence indicates a negative result. To serve as a procedural control, a colored line will always appear in the control line region indicating that proper volume of specimen has been added.

34.4 LABORATORY RECORD

Make a record of antigen–antibody reactions performed by you in the following table:

Date	Name of the antigen–antibody test performed	Observation		Teacher's signature
		Qualitative test	Quantitative test	

Enzyme-Linked Immunosorbent Assay

35.1 AIM

To familiarize the students with the principle and different methods of performing enzyme-linked immunosorbent assay (ELISA).

35.2 LEARNING OUTCOME

After this exercise, the students know the principle, different types of ELISA test and can perform the experiments independently if the facilities are available.

35.3 PURPOSE

ELISA is a widely-used method for qualitative detection and/or quantitative determination of different molecules (e.g. a bacterial, viral or fungal antigen, a hormone or drug, antibodies, etc.) in a fluid. It is also known as enzyme immunoassay or EIA.

35.4 PRINCIPLE

In ELISA, **for antigen detection,** specific antibodies that have been prepared against the particular antigen are used. Monoclonal antibodies are often used. **For detecting antibody**, specific antigen is used. Steps involved in ELISA are binding of the desired molecule on a solid phase, blocking the remaining solid matrix, labeling with a enzyme labeled molecule, adding the substrate for the enzyme and colorimetric detection of the product (Fig. 35.1).

35.5 MATERIAL REQUIRED FOR ELISA

Test Sample

Test samples containing pure antigen are usually pipetted onto the plate at a final concentration of less than 2 µg/ml. Pure solutions are not essential, but as a guideline, over 3% of the protein in the test sample should be the target protein (antigen). Antigen protein concentration should not be over 20 µg/ml as this will saturate most of the available sites on the microtitre plate.

Ensure the samples contain the antigen at a concentration that is within the detection range of the antibody.

Buffers and Reagents

Coating buffer [100 mM bicarbonate/carbonate buffer]: Antigen or antibody should be diluted in coating buffer to immobilize them to the wells:

ELISA

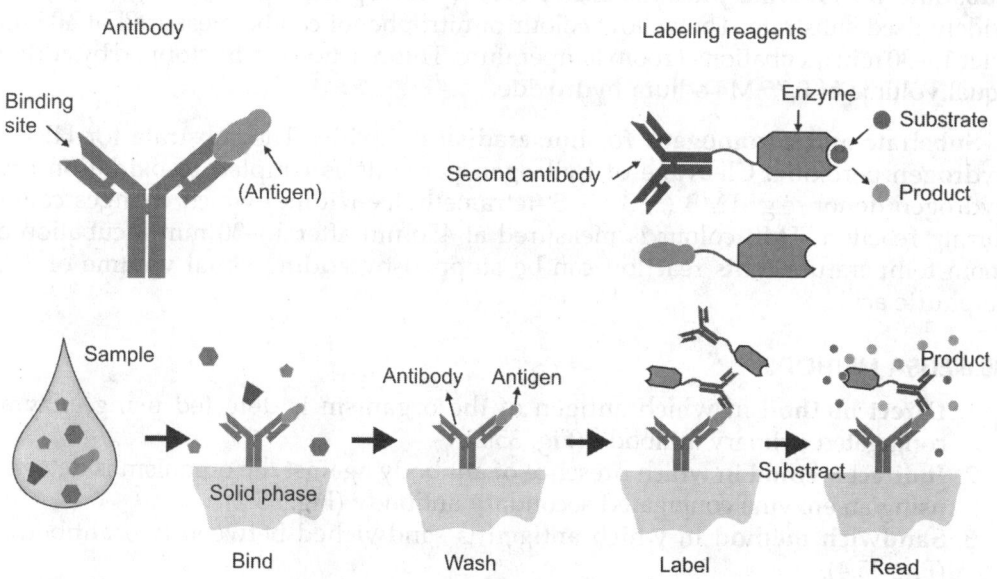

Fig. 35.1: Steps for performing ELISA

Composition of coating buffer
- 3.03 g sodium carbonate.
- 6.0 g sodium bicarbonate.
- 1000 ml distilled water.
- pH 9.6.

Blocking solution: Commonly used blocking agents are 1% BSA, serum, non-fat dry milk, casein, gelatin in PBS, etc.

Blocking Buffer (Phosphate Buffered Saline (PBS))
Composition of blocking buffer
- 1.16 g disodium hydrogen phosphate,
- 0.1 g potassium chloride.
- 0.1 g tripotassium phosphate,
- 4.0 g sodium chloride.
- 500 ml distilled water.
- pH 7.4.

Wash solution: Usually PBS or Tris-buffered saline (pH 7.4) with detergent such as 0.05% (v/v) Tween 20 (TBST).

Antibody dilution buffer: Primary and secondary antibody are diluted in 1× blocking solution to reduce non-specific binding.

Enzyme: Although many different types of enzymes have been used for detection, horse radish peroxidase (HRP) and alkaline phosphatase (ALP) are the two widely used enzymes employed in ELISA assay.

Substrate

Substrate for alkaline phosphatase: p-NPP (p-nitrophenyl-phosphate) is the most widely used substrate. The yellow colour of nitrophenol can be measured at 405 nm after 15–30 min incubation at room temperature. This reaction can be stopped by adding equal volume of 0.75 M sodium hydroxide.

Substrate and chromogens for horseradish peroxide: The substrate for HRP is hydrogen peroxide. Cleavage of hydrogen peroxide is coupled to oxidation of a hydrogen donor, e.g. TMB (3, 3′, 5, 5′-tetramethylbenzidine) which changes colour during reaction. TMB colour is measured at 450 nm after 15–30 min incubation at room temperature. This reaction can be stopped by adding equal volume of 2 M sulphuric acid.

35.6 ELISA METHODS

1. **Direct method** in which antigen of the organism is detected using enzyme conjugated primary antibody (Fig. 35.2).
2. **Indirect method** in which presence of antibody against the organism is detected using an enzyme conjugated secondary antibody (Fig. 35.2).
3. **Sandwich method** in which antigen is sandwiched between two antibodies (Fig. 35.4).

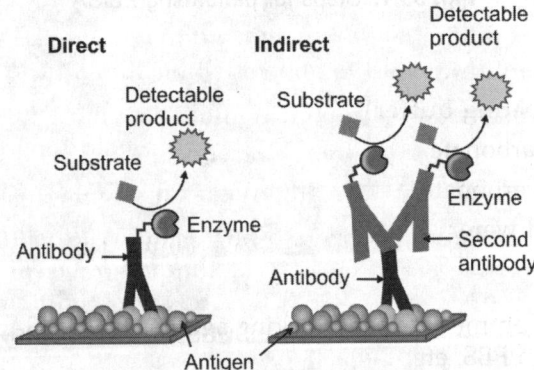

Fig. 35.2: Direct ELISA and indirect ELISA

35.6.1 Direct Method

a. Coating antigen to microtitre plate

1. Dilute the antigen in carbonate buffer to a final concentration of 20 µg/ml. Coat the wells of a PVC microtiter plate with the antigen by pipeting 50 µl of the antigen dilution in the top wells of the 96 well microtitre plate. Dilute down the plate as required.
2. Cover the plate with an adhesive plastic and incubate for 2 hours at room temperature, or at 4°C overnight.
3. Remove the coating solution and wash the plate twice by filling the wells with 200 µl PBS. Remove the solutions or washes by flicking the plate over a sink followed by patting the plate on a paper towel/blotting paper.

b. Blocking

1. Block the remaining protein-binding sites in the coated wells by adding 200 µl blocking buffer [usually 5% non-fat dry milk in PBS, per well or 1% bovine serum albumin (BSA)].

2. Cover the plate with an adhesive plastic and incubate for at least 2 hours at room temperature or overnight at 4°C.
3. Wash the plate twice with PBS.

c. Incubation with the antibody

1. Add 100 µl of the antibody, diluted at the optimal concentration (according to the manufacturer's instructions) in blocking buffer immediately before use.
2. Cover the plate with an adhesive plastic and incubate for 2 hours at room temperature or overnight at 4°C.
3. Wash the plate four times with PBS.

d. Detection

1. Dispense 100 µl (or 50 µl) of the substrate solution per well with a multichannel pipette or a multipipette.
2. After sufficient colour development (if it is necessary) add 100 µl of stop solution to the wells.
3. Read the absorbance (optical density) of each well with a plate reader.

Note: Some enzyme substrates are considered hazardous (potential carcinogens), therefore always handle the reagents with care and wear gloves.

e. Analysis of data: Prepare a standard curve from the data produced from the serial dilutions with concentration on the x axis (log scale) vs absorbance on the y axis (linear). Interpolate the concentration of the sample from this standard curve. For accurate quantitative results, always compare signal of unknown samples against those of a standard curve. Standards (duplicates or triplicates) and blank must be run with each plate to ensure accuracy.

35.6.2 Indirect ELISA

1. Coat plate with antigen. Incubate for 2 hours at room temperature or at 4°C overnight.
2. Wash plates four times with PBS with 0.2% Tween 20.
3. Block with 5% serum or BSA for 2 hours at room temperature or overnight at 4°C.
4. Wash plates four times with PBS with 0.2% Tween 20.
5. Incubate with primary antibody 2 hours at room temperature or at 4°C overnight.
6. Wash plates four times with PBS with 0.2% Tween 20.
7. Add enzyme conjugated secondary antibody. Incubate for 1–2 hours at room temperature.
8. Wash plates four times with PBS with 0.2% Tween 20.
9. Add substrate.
10. Add stop solution following manufacturer's instruction.
11. Read absorbance on ELISA plate reader and analyze results.

35.6.3 Sandwich ELISA

Steps in sandwich ELISA are shown at Fig. 35.3.

1. Incubate with coating antibody in bicarbonate buffer overnight 4°C (step 1 in Fig. 35.3).
2. Wash plates four times with PBS with 0.2% Tween 20.
3. Block with 5% serum or BSA for 2 hours at room temperature or overnight 4°C.
4. Add sample to wells and dilute down the plate (step 2 in Fig. 35.3)

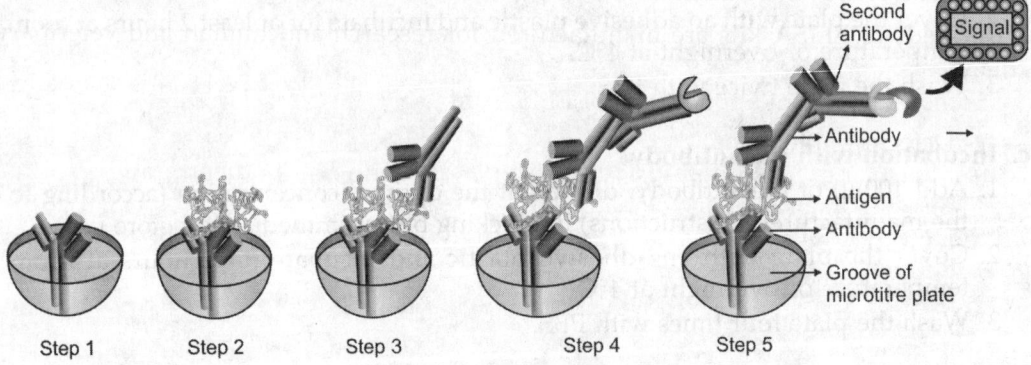

Fig. 35.3: Steps in sandwich ELISA

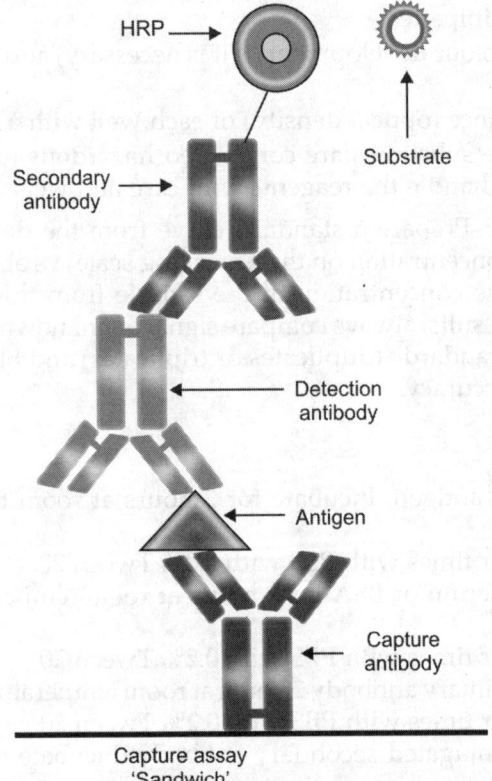

Fig. 35.4: Sandwich ELISA

5. Wash plates four times with PBS with 0.2% Tween 20.
6. Incubate with detection antibody 2 hours at room temperature (step 3 in Fig. 35.3)
7. Incubate with enzyme conjugated secondary antibody for 30 minutes to 2 hours at room temperature (step 4 in Fig. 35.3)
8. Wash four times with PBS with 0.2% Tween 20.
9. Add substrate (step 5 in Fig. 35.3)
10. Follow manufacturer's recommendations to stop the reaction.
11. Read absorbance on ELISA plate reader and analyze results.

35.7 APPLICATIONS OF ELISA

Hundreds of ELISA kits are manufactured for research and human and veterinary diagnosis.

Some examples of applications of ELISA are:

- Detecting infections.
- Measuring "rheumatoid factors" and other autoantibodies in autoimmune diseases like lupus erythematous.
- Detection of antibody and its quantitative measurement using appropriate antigen.
- Screening donated blood for evidence of viral contamination.
- Measuring hormone levels.
- Detecting allergens in food and house dust.
- Measuring toxins in contaminated food.
- Detecting illicit drugs, e.g. cocaine, marijuana, etc.

Polymerase Chain Reaction Technology

36.1 AIM

To educate the students about the polymerase chain reaction (PCR) technology.

36.2 LEARNING OUTCOME

The students understand the principle and purpose of using PCR technology and can carry out the procedure in the laboratories where the facilities exist.

36.3 PURPOSE

Polymerase chain reaction technology is used to increase the number of a particular DNA sequence exponentially from a single or a few copies of a piece of DNA even when the source DNA is of relatively poor quality.

36.4 PRINCIPLE

The polymerase chain reaction (PCR) technology is simple, quick and inexpensive application of molecular biology using a DNA template, the required nucleotides and DNA polymerase. At its optimum temperature, the DNA polymerase can polymerize a thousand bases per minute. The bases (complementary to the template) are coupled to the primer on the 3' side [the polymerase adds deoxynucleotide triphosphates (dNTP)s from 5' to 3', reading the template from 3' to 5' side, bases are added complementary to the template].

The process is performed in an automated cycler, which can heat and cool the tubes containing the reaction mixture in a very short time.

36.5 MATERIALS REQUIRED

- Template DNA in sufficient quantity (between 0.1 and 1 µg for genomic DNA).
- dNTP (deoxynucleotide triphosphate) mix (concentration of each dNTP, i.e. deoxyadenosine triphosphate, (dATP), deoxycytidinetriphosphate, (dCTP), deoxyguanosine triphosphate (dGTP), deoxythymidinetriphophate (dTTP) in the reaction mixture is usually 200 µM).
- Polymerase chain reaction (PCR) primer.
- Taq DNA polymerase in appropriate concentration to avoid synthesis of non-specific products.
- Sterile deionised water.
- 10X PCR buffer (200 mM Tris Hcl (pH 8.4), 500 mM kcl).
- Magnesium chloride (recommended range of concentration is 1 to 3 mM, under the standard reaction conditions specified).

Characteristic Feature of PCR Primers

- 10–24 nucleotides in length.
- The Guanine cytosine (GC) content should be 40–60%.
- The primer should not be self-complementary or complementary to any other primer in the reaction mixture.
- Melting temperatures of primer pairs should not differ by more than 5°C, so that the GC content and length must be chosen accordingly.
- The annealing temperature should be about 5°C lower than the melting temperature.

Equipment

- Micropipettes
- Thermocycler
- Electrophoresis units
- Power supply units
- Photographic equipment

Many PCR machines are now available in 48-, 96- or 384-well formats. This, combined with the use of multichannel pipettes, can greatly increase the number of reactions that can be done simultaneously. If several reactions need to be simultaneously prepared, a master mix should be used as follows: water, buffer, dNTPs, primers, $MgCl_2$ and Taq DNA polymerase in a single tube. This are then aliquoted into individual tubes.

36.6 STEPS INVOLVED IN PCR TECHNOLOGY

There are three major steps in a PCR, which are repeated for 30 or 40 cycles (Fig. 36.1) These steps are

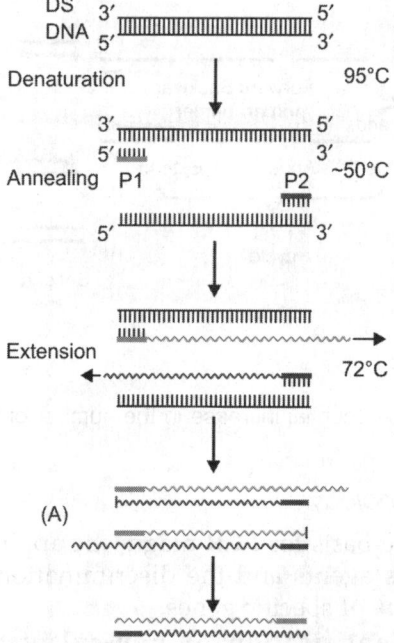

Fig. 36.1: Steps involved in PCR technology

Step 1: Denaturation at 95°C: During the denaturation, the double stranded DNA melts open to single stranded DNA, all enzymatic reactions stop. The mixture is held at the denaturation temperature for 20–30 seconds.

Step 2: Annealing at approximately 54°C for 20 to 40 seconds: During annealing, ionic bonds are constantly formed and broken between the single stranded primer and the single stranded template. Once there are a few bases built in, the ionic bond is so strong between the template and the primer, that it does not break anymore.

Step 3: Extension at 72°C: This is the ideal working temperature for the polymerase. The primers, where there are a few bases built in, already have a stronger ionic attraction to the template than the forces breaking these attractions. Primers that are on positions with no exact match get loose again (because of the higher temperature) and do not give an extension of the fragment. As a rule-of-thumb, at its optimum temperature, the DNA polymerase will polymerize a thousand bases per minute.

Step 4: Final elongation: This single step is occasionally performed at a temperature of 70–74°C for 5–15 minutes after the last PCR cycle to ensure that any remaining single-stranded DNA is fully extended.

Because both strands are copied during PCR, there is an exponential increase of the number of copies of the gene (Fig. 36.2). If there is only one copy of the wanted gene before the cycling starts, after one cycle, there will be 2 copies, after two cycles, there will be 4 copies, and three cycles will result in 8 copies and so on.

To check whether the PCR generated the anticipated DNA fragment, agarose gel electrophoresis is employed for size separation of the PCR products. The size(s) of PCR products is determined by comparison with a DNA fragments of known size, run on the gel alongside the PCR products.

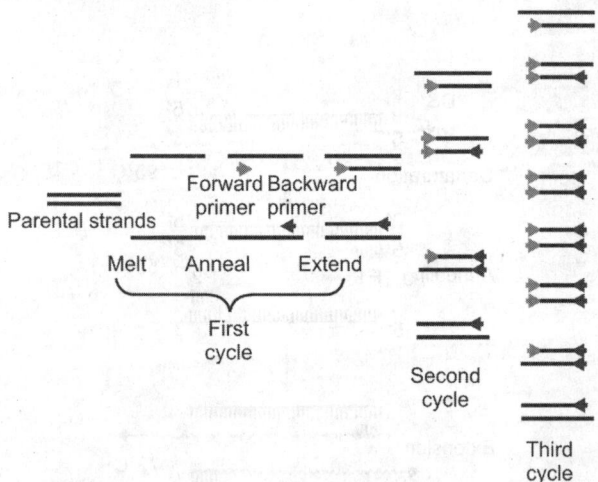

Fig. 36.2: Exponential increase in the number of DNA copies

Applications of PCR Technology

Diagnosis of diseases: The basis for PCR diagnostic applications in microbiology is the detection of infectious agents and the discrimination of non-pathogenic from pathogenic strains by virtue of specific genes.

PCR also permits **identification of non-cultivatable or slow-growing microorganisms** such as mycobacteria, anaerobic bacteria, or viruses from tissue culture assays and animal models. The high sensitivity of PCR permits virus detection soon after infection and even before the onset of disease.

PCR permits **early diagnosis of malignant diseases** such as leukemia and lymphomas, PCR assays can be performed directly on genomic DNA samples to detect translocation-specific malignant cells at a sensitivity that is at least 10,000 fold higher than that of other methods.

PCR can also be used for **selective DNA isolation** and for **DNA sequencing and amplification for forensic and archeological analysis.**

37

Automation in Clinical Microbiology Laboratory

Automation of microbiology laboratory has following advantages:

- Rapid processing of a large number of specimens.
- Accurate tracing of the specimen in subsequent processes.
- Results obtaning in a short time.
- Barcode makes every sample carrier unique.
- Eliminating of optimum use subjective variability.
- Saves media and reagents.

Lay out details of a full microbiology laboratory automation solution provided by M/S bioMérieux is illustrated in Fig. 37.1.

Other manufacturers providing microbiology laboratory automation solution are Bectin-Dickinson, Copan, Kiestra system, etc.

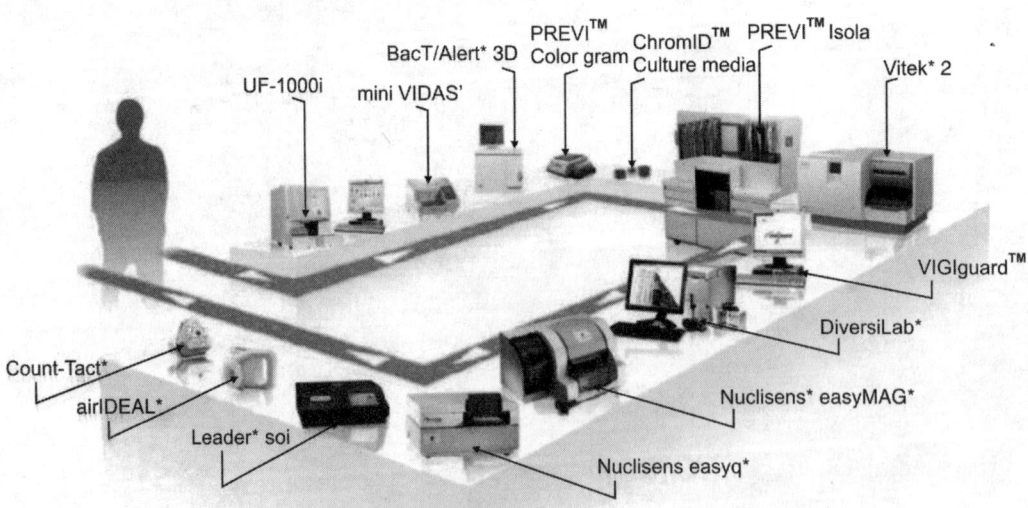

Fig. 37.1: Complete microbiology laboratory automation solutions

Some of the parameters to look for in automation at various steps are listed in Table 37.1

Table 37.1: Parameters to look for at various steps in an automated microbiology laboratory.

Area of automation	Parameters to look for
Instrument characteristics	Size. Weight of the instrument. Noise, if any. Electrical requirement. No of agar plate s/broth processed per hour Time spent in inoculation Accuracy Quality control Biosafety maintenance, etc.
Sample collection	Containers to be used. Sample size. Sample consistency and type-liquid, semiliquid, swab. Bar coding. Relationship with laboratory information system. Automated direct smear preparation at the time of sampling.
Inoculation	Selection of appropriate petridish. Inoculation of sample for semi-quantitative, quantitative evaluation. Choice of medium. Use of disposable or re-usable loop. Spreading of the inoculum to obtain well separated colonies. Accurate labeling and sorting of each inoculated medium. Automated capping/uncapping. Automated smear preparation. Automated transfer to incubator. Reading of growth on broth an agar plate. Plate inoculation for automated antimicrobial susceptibility test.
Microbial identification	Separate reagent cards for Gram-positive, Gram-negative, anaerobic and other organisms. Number of wells in each reagent card containing an individual test substrate. Substrates for measuring various metabolic activities such as acidification, alkalinization, enzyme hydrolysis, and growth in the presence of inhibitory substances. Appropriate level of oxygen transmission inside the sealed vessel.

FURTHER READING

1. Collins CH, Lyne Pm, Grange JM. Collins and Lyne's microbiology methods, 7th edition. Butterworth-Heinemann.
2. Medical Microbiology-Volumes 1 and 2, R.Cruickshank, J.P.Duguid, B.P. Marmion, R.H.A Swain 12th edition, Churchill Livingstone
3. Mackie and McCartney - Practical Medical Microbiology : Edited J.G.Collee, A.G. Fraser, B.P.Marmion, A. Simmons, Elsevier
4. Microbiology –M.J.Pelczar,R.D. Reid and E.C.S Chan , McGrawHill
5. Foundations in microbiology - Kathleen Talaro and Arther Talaro, Wm.C.Brown Publishers
6. Medical microbiology - Mims, Playfair,Roitt, Wakelin, Williams Mosby
7. Basic medical microbiology Robert F.Boyd, Bryan G.Hoerl, 4th edition , Little Brown and Company
8. Microbiology-a human perspective - Nestler, Roberts Nestler Wm C Brown Publisher 1995
9. Diagnostic microbiology -Baily and Scotts , Mosby
10. Colour atlas and textbook of diagnostic microbiology Elmer W.Koneman, S.D. Allen,M.M.Janda, P.C.Schreckenberger, W.C.Wina Jr, 4th edition, J.B.Lippincott
11. Public health mycobacteriology –a guide to the level III laboratory – Partricia T.Kent, George P.Kubica, US Department of Health and Human Services, CDC
12. Microbiology-A laboratory manual, Cuppuccino and Sherman, 7th edition, Pearson education
13. Spot tests in organic analysis – F. Fiegel and Vingeg Anger, Elsevier's Publications 1966.

WEBSITE REFERENCES

Google image sites .
bioMérieux Clinical Diagnostics website).www.pda.org/bookstore
http://supratechmicropath.com.
http://whqlibdoc.who.int/monograph/WHO_MONO_43_(chp7).pdf(ramakrishnan venkatraman medium processing of stool)
www.biolifeit.com) campylobacter agar
(www.atcc.org) reference for antibiotic sensitivity
(WWW.standardsportal.org.in/pdf/BISpresentation
www.cdc.gov transport of specimen
(www.atcc.org) reference for antibiotic sensitivity
www.icmsf.org/ ICMSF microorganisms and food
(http://www.who.int/lep/microbiology/en/) reporting of M.leprae staining
Cold Spring Harb Protoc.
www.pearsonhighered.com.
bloodjournal.hematologylibrary.org
http://zeiss-campus.magnet.fsu.edu
http://www.oxoid.com.
http://www.uq.edu.au.
http://armymedical.tpub.com.

Index

A

Acetone-alcohol 66
Acid alcohol 71
Acid fast staining
  principle 70–75
  procedure 70–75
Agar slope/agar slant 93
Agar stab 93
Air sampling
Albert stain I 76
Albert staining
  principle 76–77
  procedure 76–77
Albert's iodine 77
Alternaria 191
Ameba 57
Antisepsis 40
Antistreptolysin 198, 199
Aspergillus 192
Autoclave 35, 36

B

Bacteria responsible for food poisoning 179
Bacterial capsule 79
Bacterial flagella 62
Bacterial growth
  characteristics in liquid 102, 103
  stab cultures 102, 103
Basic fuchsin 66
Biosafety cabinets 18–20
Blood agar 86
Blood sample
  culture 163–166
  sensitivity 163–166
Bright field microscope 46, 47, 49–53

C

C reactive protein test 199, 200
Campylobacter blood agar 149

Candle jar 99
Carbohydrate fermentation test 109, 110
Carbol fuchsin 71
Cary Blair transport medium 148
Catalase test 124
Cerebrospinal fluid sample
  culture and sensitivity 167–171
Chemical method of sterilization 44
Chocolate agar 87
Christensen's medium 90
Ciliate (Paramecium) 57
Citrate utilization test 115, 116
Cleaning agents
  acid peroxide solution 23, 24
  aqua regia 23, 24
  base bath 23, 24
  hydrochloric acid 23, 24
  nitric acid 23, 24
Coagulase test 126, 127
Colony characteristics 103–105
Crystal violet 66

D

Dark field microscope 46, 47
Direct ELISA 211
Disinfection 40
Dropping bottle 2

E

Eijkman test 174
Electrical hazards 15,17
Electron microscope 46, 48
Epsilometer test (E-test) 130–131

F

Fecal sample 147–151
  culture 147–151
  sensitivity 147–151
Filtering flask 2, 3, 37

Flagellate (Giardia) 57
Fluorescent microscope 47, 48
Formalin-saline-ether 186, 187
Fungal infections
   lab diagnosis 195, 197
Fungus 56
Fusarium 192

G

Gas pak system 100, 101
Gelatin liquefaction test 122, 123
Gentian violet 66
Glucose broth 86
Glucose phosphate 85
Graduated pipettes 2, 3
Gram staining 65–69
   principle 65–69
   procedure 65–69
Grams iodine 66

H

Hanging drop
   preparation for bacterial motility 62–64
Hazard symbols
   chemical and reagent hazards (GHS symbol)
   16
HEPA filter 38, 44
Hot air oven 33, 34
Hugh and Leifson medium 90
Hydrogen sulphide production test 117, 118

I

Impactor 182
Impinger 182
Indirect ELISA 212
Indole test 116, 117
Inspissator 34, 35

K

Kirby-Bauer method 130–133

L

Labels 11, 12
Lawn culture 97, 98
Light microscope 46

M

MacCartney bottle 2
MacConkey agar 87, 88

MacIntosh and Filde's jar 99, 100
MacFarland standard 131
Malachite green 72
Measuring cylinder 2, 3
Mechanical hazards 15, 17
Membrane filters 37, 38, 44
Methyl red test 112, 113
Methylene blue 59, 72
Methylene blue reduction time 177
Microbiology 55, 56
   labortary automation 219, 220
Mohr pipette 2, 3
Morphology and arrangement of
   bacteria 55, 56
Most probable number (MPN) of organisms 175
Mucor 192
Müller Hinton agar 91

N

Nasopharyngeal swab
   culture 154–157
   sensitivity 154–157
Negative staining 79–81
NIH swab 185
Nitrate reduction test 119–121
Numerical aperture 50
Nutrient agar 86
Nutrient broth 85
Nutrient gelatin 123

O

Oxidase test 125, 126
Oxidative and fermentative 110, 112
   utilization of carbohydrate 110, 112

P

Packaging and transport of specimen 140
PCR technology 215, 217
Penicillium 193
Peptone water 85
Permissible limit of organisms in drinking
   water 176
Permissible number of bacteria in milk 178
Personal protective equipment 14
Petridish 2, 3
Phase contrast microscope 47
Phenylalanine deaminase test 121, 122
Pipettes 2, 25, 31
Plugging of glassware 30, 31
Pour plate 97, 98

Pus sample
  culture 152, 153
  sensitivity 152, 153

R

Resolution 50
Rheumatoid factor 201, 202
Rhizopus 193
Ringer soulation 178

S

Sabouraud's agar medium 194
Safranin 66
Sandwich ELISA 212, 213
Scanning tunneling microscope 46
Sedimentation method 186, 187
Selenite broth 149
Serological pipette 2, 3
Settle plate 181
Simmon's citrate 89
Sodium pyruvate agar 194
Sporozoa (malaria parasite) 57
Sputum sample
  culture 158–161
  sensitivity 158–161
Sterilization 40
  flaming 43
  heating to redness 42
Stoke method 130
Streak plate 96, 97
Stuart transport medium 149
Sulphuric acid 71

T

Thioglycollate broth 165
Throat swab

culture 154–157
  sensitivity 154–157
Total magnification 49
Trans-isolate (T-I) medium 168, 169
Triple sugar iron 89
Tripticase soya broth 164

U

Universal precautions 18
Urease test 118, 119
Urine
  culture 143–145
  sensitivity 143, 145

V

VDRL test 202, 203
Venkatraman-Ramakrishnan medium 150
Voges-Proskauer test 113–115

W

Wait film preparation of stool 185
Water sampling 173
WHO guideline 173
Widal test 204, 207
Wrapping of laboratory ware 30

X

Xylose-lysine deoxycholate agar 88

Y

Yeast extract agar 174

Z

Zinc sulphate floatation method 186
Zone of inhibition 133